SHIATSU

Jane Downer

Headway · Hodder & Stoughton

The publisher and author would like to thank Christina Jansen, Siobhan Chandler and Gary Ivison for the cover photograph, Julie Downer for the photographs on pages 13, 23, 27, 89, 92, 102, Roddy Paine for taking all the text photographs and Sue Tindall, Jeff Kear and James Regan for modelling for the photographs.

British Library Cataloguing in Publication Data

Downer, Jane
    Headway lifeguide: Shiatsu. – (Headway lifeguides)
    I. Title   II. Series
    615.8

ISBN 0–340–55321–9

First published 1992

© Jane Downer 1992

Typeset by Wearside Tradespools, Fulwell, Sunderland

Printed in Great Britain for the educational publishing division of Hodder & Stoughton Ltd, Mill Road, Dunton Green, Sevenoaks, Kent by Thomson Litho Ltd

CONTENTS

FOREWORD

As Shiatsu continues to grow in popularity throughout the world, there is an ever increasing demand for high quality instruction and literature on the subject. With this book, Jane Downer has helped to fulfil one of the aims of The European Shiatsu School; namely, to produce top quality written material for the beginner, which describes Shiatsu in the overall context of the healing arts as they are practised today. More than that, she has used her skills as an artist to convey the spirit of Shiatsu through more than 60 illustrations.

This beginner's guide is therefore part of an overall strategy to fulfil the requirements of all those interested in Shiatsu. This strategy pivots around developing 'grassroots' Shiatsu training courses designed to equip all interested people with the skills necessary to de-stress their friends and communicate more openly through touch; moreover, to provide these courses as locally as possible, thereby ensuring maximum accessibility and to provide clear literature on basic Shiatsu (hence this book). This complements the professional Diploma Courses offered by the European Shiatsu School and similar establishments.

Whatever your degree of interest, this book has something to say to you.

Chris Jarmey
Principal – European Shiatsu School

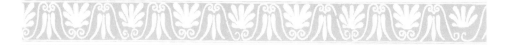

PREFACE

" Health comes from joy in life. "
Shizuto Masunaga

Energy flows within all of us and within nature. Along with the right conditions and environment it is movement of this energy that allows cleansing, repair, regeneration and growth to take place in all living things.

This movement happens naturally and continually, to the point that most people are hardly even aware of it and take it for granted.

When life energy flows smoothly, health is maintained. When something disturbs and inhibits this activity we become vulnerable to ill-health and it is eventually felt as symptoms of illness or disease.

Nobody wants ill health but unfortunately it is common to be unwell. Minor disorders and annoying symptoms are often regarded as something to be put up with and people increasingly *expect* health problems, especially as they grow old.

Illness does not usually 'just happen' to us. The problem is that we are largely unaware of the part that we play in causing our own sickness. We do not see how our health disorders are often created slowly over the years by the culmination of how we live, what we think, feel, eat, breathe, do and do not do.

The effects of harsh and traumatic life experiences clearly can be damaging to our health and well being. However a less obvious factor is the way in which every cell of our body, the very fabric of our health, is affected by our temperament, thoughts and feelings.

At some level the mind controls the activity of the body. How else can billions of cells co-operate to create and support the life of an individual? We underestimate this influence. Both mental stress, including unconscious daily negative thought patterns and emotional attitudes, and the build up of toxins in the body adversely affect and block our life energy. This encourages poor health.

What we need to realise is that under most circumstances germs, bacteria and viruses have little power to cause illness in strong and healthy people. Of course, we are vulnerable to extreme situations but it is the condition within the individual which is the deciding factor in a person's susceptibility to sickness and infection.

Generally speaking germs can only take advantage of a state of weakness in the body. After all, we live in intimate contact with millions of assorted micro-organisms and the majority of people still enjoy reasonable, if not good health most of the time.

Ill health can be viewed in a positive way. It is a signal that your body is in a state of disharmony and it confronts you with the need to change if healing is to take place. This change may be simple, like the need for rest, or it may involve a more drastic alteration of life style, diet or attitude.

True healing requires that the whole person be treated and not the disease, germ or virus. This healing occurs from within and the individual has to become actively involved in the process.

A person's attitude is significant in this. Most importantly, the tendency to blame others and outside circumstances needs to be changed to the desire to assume self responsibility through self reflection. We need to recognise and accept the part that we play in whatever happens to us. We have a responsibility for our health and how we feel and we have the power and means to help ourselves through preventative health practices. Shiatsu offers one of the many means by which we can take care of ourselves and maintain good health.

INTRODUCTION

> **❝** *Touch is a mystical sense relating to spirit, soul and body.* **❞**
> Ida Mingle

Shiatsu is for everyone. No special equipment or qualifications are needed for you to start save your own desire and a feeling of care and tenderness towards yourself and others.

Shiatsu is a Japanese physical therapy. As you practise and study it in depth its ability to help in relieving and curing many disorders and ailments becomes apparent.

Giving Shiatsu is a wonderful way to show your love to family and friends. It is enjoyable, relaxing and deeply fulfilling, and as a bonus it promotes good health, well being and vitality. Moreover, when you give to others in this way you also benefit yourself. Through understanding and practising Shiatsu, your own potential will in time increasingly unfold and open you more fully to life and its many opportunities.

Over the last 20 years Shiatsu has developed in the West in a remarkable way. It is now widely practised in the private health sector and its benefits are increasingly being officially recognised and used in hospitals and institutions.

The importance of touch

Touch is the essential factor in Shiatsu. Given with tenderness and care it nourishes us emotionally and spiritually, and enhances our sense of self worth. Touch given in this way also affects the body, stimulating circulation, promoting relaxation and a feeling of well being.

Quite naturally we touch and hug each other to show love and support and to reassure, soothe and ease pain. We heal ourselves every day when we instinctively hold and rub our own sore muscles and tense areas.

Touch is a very direct form of communication which is received through the skin, the largest and most sensitive organ of the body. The skin is in fact developed from the same cell layer as the nervous system in the growing embryo and it contains a huge amount of nerve cells.

Our thoughts, motives and intent, in other words 'how' we touch, deeply influences the effect it has on someone. Used positively touch enhances the body's own self healing abilities and it is this quality that is essential to Shiatsu.

Understanding Shiatsu

The principles of Shiatsu have been practised for centuries in the Orient although the name Shiatsu only came into common use less than a hundred years ago.

Shiatsu is a Japanese word translated literally as 'finger' (*shi*) 'pressure' (*atsu*). As well as fingers practitioners also use their thumbs, whole hand, elbows, knees and feet to press, massage and manipulate the body.

Over the years Shiatsu has evolved into various forms which emphasise different aspects of approach. Some forms emphasise Acupressure which requires the precise use of tsubos. Other forms are concerned primarily with pressure to, and manipulation of, the channels. Shiatsu is strengthened by this diversity and richness of expression, all of which have grown out of the understanding and theory of traditional oriental medicine.

How it works

The practice of Shiatsu basically expands upon the natural qualities and characteristics of touch, which it combines with the ancient theory of Oriental Medicine. This is based on the observation that the body and mind are interrelated and function as one. The understanding is that life energy, known as 'Ki', flows throughout the body along a network of non-physical pathways or channels, also known as the meridians.

When energy flow is consistently blocked, weak or excessively strong in any of these Ki channels it will show in the body as symptoms of disease. In other words your good health is dependent on balanced and freely flowing life energy. This is a fundamental idea in Shiatsu.

Ki is also stimulated by touch and Shiatsu techniques are designed to help remove blockages and balance Ki flow. The channels are activated in a general way or more precisely by pressing particular points or 'tsubos' located along their length.

The function of channels and flow of Ki is a more subtle expression of the body's sensitivity than the nervous system, in the same way that the activity of the nervous system is more subtle than that of blood and circulation. Ki energy and the nervous system do, however, interrelate and affect each other. When the body is touched with love and care both these systems respond in a deep way that can bring harmony and balance to the whole body.

Prevention is best

The real strength of Shiatsu lies in its use as a preventative therapy.

The day to day disturbances and minor disorders in our health and well being such as headaches, indigestion, constipation or diarrhoea, fatigue, stress, depression, back pain, sinus congestion and so on can all be treated with Shiatsu. It is particularly effective when used in conjunction with adjustments to diet and lifestyle.

Of course we can live with these symptoms and often do so. However when left unchecked and untreated for years, these small complaints can easily become chronic conditions and become hard to live with. At this stage complete recovery can be difficult and very costly to achieve.

Given regularly Shiatsu will build and strengthen your body and continually help it to heal itself.

East and West

The approach to and understanding of health and medicine in the East may seem strange to many of us in the West, but the idea of the integration and interrelatedness of everything in the Universe is not new.

This century has seen the rediscovery of ancient wisdoms, understanding and practices. Many of these are in the field of health care and medicine. They involve the use of massage, Shiatsu, acupuncture, medicinal herbs, moxibustian, various forms of exercise, Martial Arts, yoga, approaches to diet, fasting, body cleansing programmes . . . the list is long. Although many seem to come from Eastern traditions, more fundamentally this knowledge represents the re-emergence of a way of perceiving, thinking and understanding that is not defined by categories with boundaries.

The approaches of both intuition and logic are like two sides of the same coin. In reality intuition is a quality of the right side of the brain, with logic being a product of the left side. One needs the other to function truly.

The great opportunity and challenge of today is in understanding and working with the complementary nature of both visions.

HOW TO USE THIS BOOK

Shiatsu is essentially something you learn by doing it.

Reading about Shiatsu can give you an idea of what to expect and an understanding of how it works. But it cannot teach you the quality of touch, how to handle and move a person or develop your sensitivity.

It is with the experience of actually giving Shiatsu that you learn this. Consequently, this book is designed as a practical guide to giving Shiatsu. It emphasises the 'how to' of giving a treatment.

The first part of the book deals with the use of 'tools', Shiatsu technique and your approach to your partner and to giving a treatment.

Shiatsu theory and understanding is put in the second half of the book. It is there for your reference and study as you practise and develop your Shiatsu.

Shiatsu has a lot to offer – enjoy it!

1

BASIC TECHNIQUE

Use of hara

In the Orient the 'hara' is seen as the energy centre of man and woman and the point of balance physically, emotionally and spiritually. Hara is a Japanese word meaning belly or abdomen; the area of the hara is from the tip of the breast bone to the pubis. Three finger widths down from the navel indicates the centre point of the hara known as the 'tanden'.

Many people have their centre of gravity situated higher than at tanden. In the West this is common and visible in the modern western life style. For example, furniture is designed to raise people off the ground, and windows are usually built high. The accepted ideal of a good male physique is a big chest with a small waist, and high heels have long been fashionable for women. Mind and thought are generally valued above intuition and feeling.

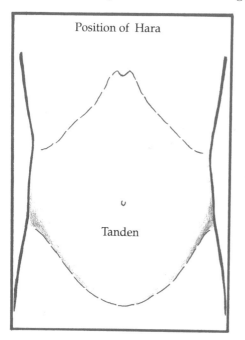

Position of Hara

Tanden

Activating your hara (see pages 29, 34), and making the pelvis your centre of gravity connects you to the ground through your legs and feet. Being 'grounded' means you have a far greater awareness of your own body and contact with intuition than you would have with your awareness concentrated on thoughts and mind (see pages 29, 133). Movement which comes from your hara and not just from your arms and shoulders naturally has co-ordination and is more relaxed.

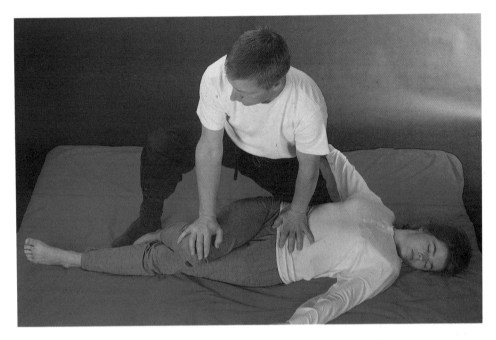

This is important when giving Shiatsu as it helps you to give treatments without becoming tired; indeed you can feel energised after giving good Shiatsu.

Giving a treatment

In Shiatsu your body is your 'tool' and hands, fingers, thumbs, elbows, knees and feet are all used in giving a treatment. Various amounts of pressure and types of stretching form the basis of Shiatsu technique along with holding and ways of rubbing, shaking, kneading and pounding the body.

The treatment is given clothed on the floor. This allows you a maximum range of movement around your partner and makes it easy for you to place their arms, legs and body in whatever position is needed.

Make physical contact with your partner slowly and gently. In touching him or her it is essential for you to use your own sensitivity to know and feel how much pressure to give, and for how long.

Approach

Each person is individual in their requirement depending on their age and condition. In Shiatsu the touch, amount of pressure and manner in which it is given and its consequent effect can vary greatly, even though the actual technique used may be similar.

There are two fundamental approaches to a treatment; that of tonifying or building up energy when it is low and that of dispersing over-active or blocked energy when it is excessive. Your initial overall observation of a person and your intuition will tell you something of how they feel and indicate the type of treatment to give them.

When energy is low and weak through illness or because of age, a gentle treatment is needed, using less physical pressure and more of the holding techniques and palm healing. This has the effect of supporting and tonifying the body as it strengthens and increases Ki energy. This condition of low or empty Ki is called 'kyo'. The opposite condition of fullness or apparent excess Ki is known as 'jitsu' (see page 124).

Generally the condition of larger and stronger people with more muscle form and stiffness is considered jitsu and a more vigorous Shiatsu is required to move their energy. Increased pressure and rubbing, rocking and shaking techniques can be used to activate Ki which has stagnated, causing tension and pain in the body.

Observing a person as a whole can indicate whether their predominant condition is kyo or jitsu. However both states will be present and a combination of both approaches is commonly used in one treatment.

Giving pressure

Basic pressure

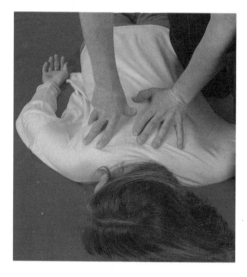

The standard type of pressure used in Shiatsu is given perpendicular to the body and held steady, without moving. Initially your touch should be light and be increased slowly when you feel that your partner becomes receptive to your pressure as her muscles relax. Work at her speed without forcing and you will find that a surprisingly strong and penetrating pressure can be achieved and still be comfortable. Hold for some seconds and release gradually when you sense a response in her energy (see pages 16, 17).

Your partner may experience pain from your pressure, but it should still feel 'good' and be beneficial. Sharp or uncomfortable pain indicate that your touch is inappropriate and should be adjusted.

Leaning in

Shiatsu should be effortless. The pressure applied and strength of treatment is *not* given with the muscle power of your arms and shoulders, but by using your body weight and 'leaning into' a person.

To do this you must remain balanced with your hands and

shoulders relaxed and let your arms support you as you move your own weight forward over your partner. There is no 'trying' or 'doing' in this; you simply allow your body weight and gravity to do the work for you.

1 Kneel facing your partner with your hands relaxed and moulded to the contours of her body. Keep your elbows firm but not locked as you shift your body weight forward. Allow yourself to be supported by your arms and by your partner. For lighter pressure kneel closer to her body.

To increase your pressure come up to your knees, so that more of your weight will be supported as you 'lean into' your partner.

At all times, give pressure with your arms perpendicular to the body.

2 Lean into which ever part of your body you are using as your 'tool' to give Shiatsu, for instance, elbows, knees, feet.

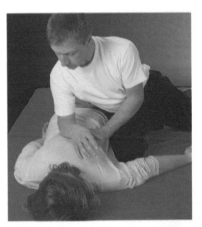

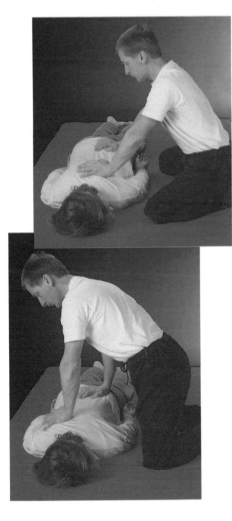

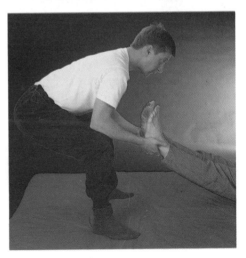

3 In a similar way, you can 'lean back' from a person and use your body weight to extend a stretch or lift a person rather than pulling with your arms. Hold your partner and lean your weight back to the extent that they can support your weight.

By letting your partner support or anchor you in this way even a small person can give effective Shiatsu to someone very large without becoming tired. You can give and maintain strong pressure and lift heavy people in an easy and a relaxed way.

Equally a soft and more gentle treatment can be given simply by controlling the use of your body weight. Care and awareness is needed as this can be a powerful way to work. You must be centred, move from your hara (see page 29) and be conscious of your partner's needs and condition.

Breathing

You need to be relaxed and feel comfortable as you give Shiatsu. Tune into the rhythm of your partner's breathing and let it influence your movements. A basic rule is to apply pressure as both of you breathe out. This is the emptying and eliminating part of the breathing cycle. As a person exhales, their body lets go and relaxes, opening to allow your touch to penetrate deeply.

The space between the out breath and the next in breath is when complete relaxation can take place in a person, so it is extremely beneficial to hold the pressure during this period, releasing it as your partner breathes in again.

Giving pressure on the out breath is especially important when you are working on the chest, hara and back areas of the body, where the physical activity of the lungs is easily felt. Inhalation could be made uncomfortable by unyielding pressure in these regions. When you want to hold a point for longer than one breath, slightly ease the weight of the pressure on your partner to allow them a comfortable inhalation, and then increase it again as they exhale.

Some techniques need specific breathing and you can direct your partner and tell the person to 'breathe in' when this is appropriate.

Keeping contact

Keep both hands in contact with your partner as much as you can during a treatment. Let one hand be more active and stimulate the points and channels while the other hand rests on the body and supports it.

Generally the moving hand goes out from the supporting hand, which holds and gives even pressure. This kind of holding pressure feels safe and is calming, producing a feeling of wholeness in your partner which

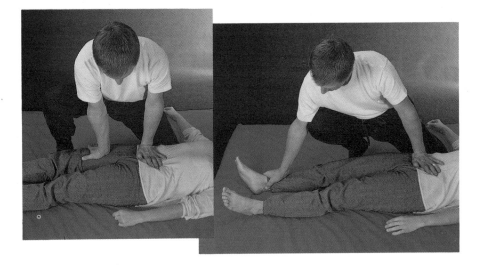

allows her to open up and relax more deeply. Holding with a steady pressure allows you the opportunity to feel the true condition of that part of the body more clearly. The work of your active hand will invigorate Ki activity and with both hands working together, Ki moves to balance itself. When this takes place, with practice, you will begin to sense the subtle changes in your partner's energy . This can be felt as a connection between both your hands. At each point your active hand moves to allow time for this connection to take place. It's as though your two hands become one with a flow of energy between them. When this happens your partner will also experience the two points of your touch as one and the effect and benefit of your Shiatsu will become more profound.

Your knee, elbow or forearm can be used instead of the active hand and at times they can also replace the support hand.

The continuity and flow of your treatment is important. Let part of your body always be in contact with your partner as you change position so that he or she knows where you are. It is also important to avoid sudden movements that might startle.

Correct position

Have your knees apart and be centred in your hara. This is your foundation. Keep your back straight and shoulders relaxed and move your weight from your hips. Let your arms be firm yet not locked and your hands relaxed as they rest on your partner and give pressure. Keep your belly and pelvic area soft and facing your partner (see 'Leaning in' photographs).

Use of tools

There are many different ways to use the 'tools' of Shiatsu.

A general rule of approach is to work from the broad to the specific by seeing your partner as a whole before concentrating on the details. This means that usually the whole hand, forearm, knee or foot is used to prepare an area before a more precise and penetrating pressure is given by the thumbs, finger tips or point of an elbow. For example, you can 'palm' down the back of the legs before tracing specific channels more exactly using thumb pressure. In giving a treatment be creative and vary the techniques and contrast your positions by using holding and more passive forms between active ones. In this way you will balance your own movements and not tire so easily.

Hands

Hands are your most versatile 'tool' in Shiatsu. The thumb and palm are most commonly used to give pressure along with your fingers, knuckles and the side of the hand.

The hands must be relaxed and act as a channel for the weight of your body to 'pass through' into your partner. This weight is felt as pressure. They also need to be receptive and responsive to your partner and gather information for you that will help you to give a treatment specifically suited to her condition and needs.

Elbows, knees and feet are also employed and give a stronger more dispersed action. These need to be used in a relaxed way. With practice they can be skilfully controlled to apply pressure with great senstivity.

Thumbs

Thumbs are a convenient size for stimulating tsubos. Pressure is usually given with the pads and sometimes with the tips.

1 Keep your hands relaxed as you use the ball of your thumb to give

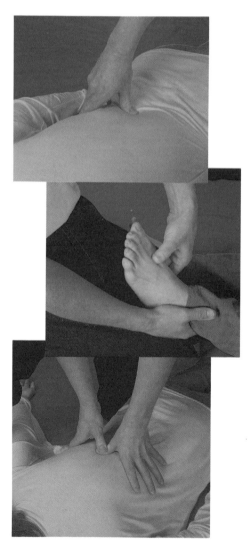

pressure. Extend your other fingers and rest them on your partner to give you support. This will also be reassuring to her.

2 The tip of your thumb gives a sharper pressure and can be used when you want more precision or to reach smaller areas.

3 Two thumbs can be used together placed side by side. For example, down each side of the spine or on top of each other to give increased pressure.

Fingers

Fingers give a lighter pressure and can be used for more delicate work such as on the face, in the abdomen, and on small children and babies. Your fingers can be used individually, together or one on top of the other.

1 Use the index and the middle finger opened as shown. This is especially good for working down each side of the spine of small children and frail people.

2 Give pressure with the tips of the index, middle and ring fingers held close together or slightly apart. This is good for treating the abdomen and working down each side of the breast bone, around the skull and over the face.

3 Squeeze, knead and hold parts of the body between your thumb and index finger (and middle finger if necessary). Use this technique on fingers, toes, and also on tense muscles such as those along the top of the shoulders and down the side and back of neck.

4 Press, knead, rub or vibrate with the pads of all your fingers and thumb. This is a good way to stimulate the skull and also other areas of the body where muscles are tight and need some loosening before deeper pressure can be given.

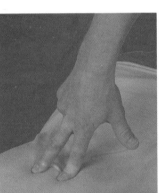

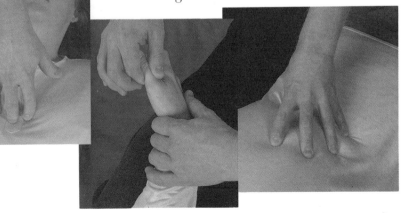

Palms

When relaxed the palm of the hand provides a good soothing pressure. It should rest on the body and mould to its contours. The pressure that you apply comes from your body weight and it should feel natural without any unnecessary pressing or forcing (see page 14). This use of your hand is called 'palming'.

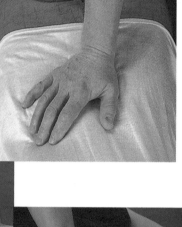

1 Palm pressure can be used very effectively on the strong areas of the body like the back, thighs and upper arms.

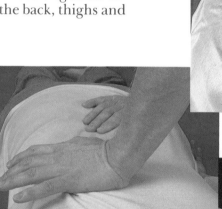

2 Palms can be used in a soft, sensing way when working on the hara.

3 For a more penetrating pressure emphasis the heel of your hand. The heels of both your hands can be used together, to stretch an area of your partner's body, for example the back.

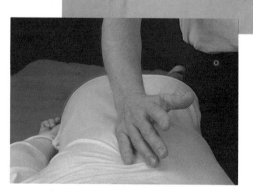

4 For more precision use the outside edge of your hand. This is effective in pressing the soft area of the abdomen under the rib cage and by the groin. It can also be used with a 'sawing' movement up and down the muscles either side of the spine.

Knuckles and fists

You can give steady and direct pressure when using your knuckles or fists to give Shiatsu. It is important to keep the bent fingers and whole hand relaxed and comfortable, yet firm. Stay well balanced by having your attention in your hara, and your knees wide apart. Use your body's weight to apply pressure, with your other hand supporting and stabilising you.

1 Use your thumb to support your index finger knuckle to give precise and penetrating pressure.

2 For more dispersed pressure use the knuckles of all four fingers, supported by your thumb.

3 The knuckles can be used in a rolling motion. This action is good on large muscle areas like the buttocks and also on the soles of the feet.

4 Form a fist without tensing your fingers, to apply powerful and direct pressure.

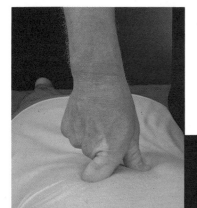

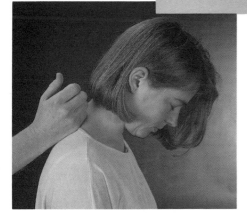

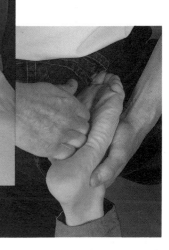

Elbows

Be aware of the sharpness of your elbow and use it in a natural non-forcing way, with your wrist and hand relaxed. The angle of your elbow affects the degree and type of pressure it can give and you can alter this as you feel changes in your partner's body. Steady your elbow with your other hand if necessary.

1 An open elbow will give a softer type of pressure.

2 A more acutely bent elbow will give a sharper pressure.

3 Use the flat forearm to treat a larger area.

both of your hands as you give pressure with your knee.

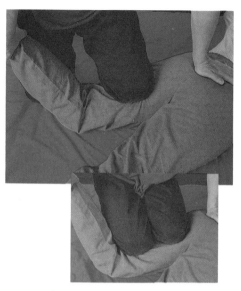

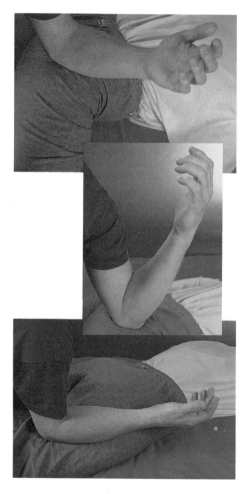

Use knee pressure mainly on the muscular parts of the body such as buttocks, legs and back.

Feet

Used with dexterity and awareness feet can give a complete Shiatsu treatment. Quite quickly you can work around your partner's body to loosen and relax her in a general way before giving a more specific treatment.

Press, push and rock your partner's body with one foot.

Knees

Knees are more powerful than the elbows and must be used with attention and control. Support and regulate your body's weight with

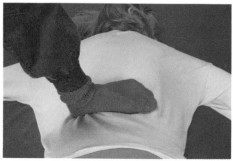

Ways of working

Balance

Giving Shiatsu on the floor means that you need a degree of flexibility and fitness to be able to move comfortably and to adjust your partner. It is important that you can work without becoming tired, even when you give many Shiatsu treatments one after each other.

The secret of this is for you to be constantly in balance as you move. When you give Shiatsu you will be moving on all fours and crawling most of the time. Watch how a baby does this. Naturally their belly is soft and hangs down, their back is relaxed and their diagonally opposite arms and legs move together. As you give Shiatsu, move with the same naturalness and balance. When you move your active hand to give pressure, at the same time move your diagonally opposite knee. Have a feeling of yourself crawling like a baby. Even when you are remaining in one place to work, shift your weight from knee to knee and echo the movement of your hands.

The diagonal type of movement of your limbs has a coordinating effect on the right and left hemispheres of the brain. It creates balance in your body and mind and it is called 'cross patterning'. This is our natural and balanced way to do things and moving like this allows you to work continuously in a relaxed way without getting too tired.

Perpendicular pressure

This is the classic way of touching in Shiatsu. (See page 14)

When a person is tense and their muscles tight, other methods of using touch can be incorporated into the treatment to encourage relaxation, movement of Ki and healing.

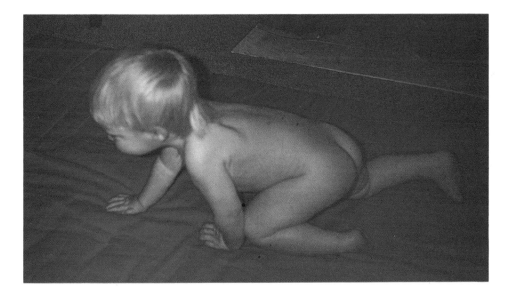

Rocking

This is one of the quickest ways to relax a person. Use your hands or feet to give small pushes to your partner, letting her own speed of 'rocking back' determine the rhythm. Any part of the body can be rocked to loosen it. A foot used on the hips and buttocks will very effectively relax the whole body.

Shaking

Gently shaking a person's arms and legs will encourage them to 'let go' and release any tension. This will stimulate and increase movement of energy in the body.

Kneading

Muscles and areas that are tight can be kneaded in a circular movement with your thumb and squeezed between your thumb and fingers. This is very effective when used on the muscles along the top of the shoulders and down the side and back of the neck.

In doing this circulation is encouraged and stiffness and pain relieved.

Pounding

Pounding quickly and rhythmically with your fingers, palm or fist is revitalising and stimulating to your partner.

It should be light and done in a way that feels easy and comfortable.

Stretching

All parts of the body can be stretched and joints bent to stimulate the channels and tsubos.

Stretching also increases mobility and circulation.

Holding and palm healing

With your support hand resting on your partner, place your other hand lightly on her body or hold it just above the skin surface. As you do this be relaxed and 'centred' in your hara and concentrate on sending energy out through the palm of your hand into your partner. You can visualise this healing energy as a stream of light coming from your hara, up your body and down your arm. Or see yourself empty and able to receive energies streaming down from above, flowing through you and emerging through your hands into your partner. At the same time encourage your partner to be centred in her hara and to become aware of receiving healing. Stay like this for some time.

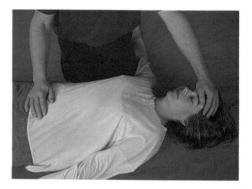

Palm healing can be used at any time, especially over very painful areas, for instance, burns and open wounds, and with illnesses such as cancer.

A final word

The form of your treatment depends on the condition of your partner, so you must allow the person to dictate what you do and the pace at which you work. Watch for indications of discomfort and be aware of changes in facial expression and of any muscles tensing. This information is important and you should be willing to alter your technique at any time during the treatment as you learn more about your partner. Ask them how it feels and encourage feedback on your treatment whilst you are doing it if necessary and also afterwards. This will help you learn and gain confidence and a sense of what is right pressure and good touch. With practice your sensitivity will develop. As you become more fully centred in your hara and become 'grounded' a feeling of 'rightness' will register in your body when your touch is effective, even as a physical sensation. You will intuitively come to know what is needed.

Preliminary exercises

The shift from being centred in your head to being centred in your hara is important and not always easy to do at first.

To give effective Shiatsu it is important to be aware of your movements and to be sensitive as you give your partner pressure. Practise these preliminary exercises so that you begin to get a feeling for what it means to move from your hara before you try to use any of the techniques.

Shifting your weight

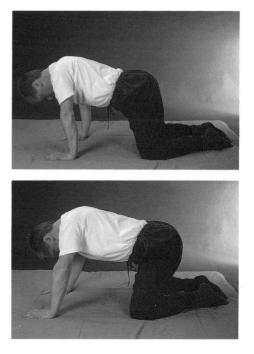

1 Position yourself on all fours. Let your spine relax and slightly dip, your head hang and your belly soften.

2 Breathe deeply through your nose. Centre yourself.

3 As you breathe out, slowly shift your weight forward onto your hands. Rest like this for some breaths and feel the concentration of your weight through your arms.

4 Then gently ease your weight back onto your knees and again hold and relax this position. Sense the difference in your balance.

5 Repeat this 2 or 3 times, moving on your exhalation.

6 Now roll your weight to one side and then to the other in a similar way . . .

7 . . . and onto one hand or the other and one knee or the other.

Move slowly and very consciously. Be aware of the feeling in your hara as you move and notice the sensation in your body when you shift your weight.

As you relax more fully let the movements flow into each other with a circular motion.

Shifting your weight with a partner

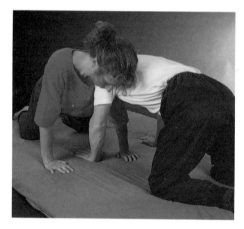

1 Face your partner on all fours and put your right shoulder to her right shoulder.

2 Centre yourself and move in the way previously described in harmony and unison with your partner. As she sways her weight forward, ease your weight back and so on in a give and take way, keeping your shoulders always in contact.

3 Repeat with your left shoulder to her left shoulder.

Do this in a gently flowing way with no competition and no forcing. Let your own sensitivities to each other make the movements like a dance.

Baby walking

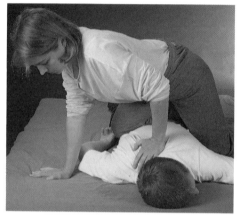

1 Be on all fours, centred and relaxed.

2 Slowly begin to crawl around the room. Keep your hara soft, spine flexible and head hanging.

3 Crawl like this as much as you can, with awareness and attention on your movement. Practise this frequently.

4 Then have a friend lie flat on the floor, face down. Continue your crawling up and over him. Approach him from different angles being careful to adjust your movements to suit the different parts of his body that you put weight on. Always avoid the back of his knees.

5 Stay relaxed and centred in your hara as you do this.

If no bodies are available then crawl over cushions and other convenient objects.

2

STEP BY STEP GUIDE

> **❝ *The way to do is to be.* ❞**
> Lau Tzu

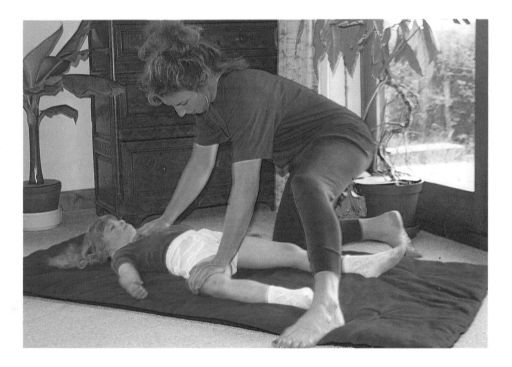

Preparation

Shiatsu is given with your partner clothed and lying or sitting on the floor or sometimes sitting in a chair.

What you require

No special equipment is needed to give Shiatsu and oils are not used. Both you and your partner should feel comfortable and warm.

Equipment

You will need something for your partner to lie on, for example, a sleeping bag, folded blanket, a futon, or a thin foam mattress covered with a sheet. A well carpeted floor will provide increased softness. If your floor is hard you may need extra layers of padding. Also have some cushions at hand in case you need them to support your partner during the treatment.

The environment

The room in which you give Shiatsu should be clean and clear of unnecessary objects. You need enough space for comfortable movement around your partner when she is lying down. Make sure the room is draft free and warm, with soft lighting that does not shine into your partner's eyes. In some instances quiet and gentle music can help a person relax, but consider your use of it as it can be intrusive. Finally, unplug the telephone – any interruptions will be a disturbance.

Clothing

Shiatsu differs from most other forms of massage in that a person receives it fully clothed. The clothes should be light, loose and comfortable to allow a full range of movement and should preferably be made of natural fibre such as cotton. Before the treatment your partner should take off her shoes, watch and any jewelery.

Likewise when you give Shiatsu you need to wear loose, comfortable clothing and remember that you will get warmer as you work. Remove your watch and any jewelery and most important, make sure your hands are clean and finger nails short.

Centering, grounding and hara

The effectiveness of your Shiatsu treatment primarily depends on your contact with yourself and your awareness in the present, or 'centering'. Technique is also important but, on its own, without your focused attention on your partner and within yourself, it is an empty shell.

The idea of centering is fundamental to all forms of Martial Arts, meditation and sports. In fact, it is an essential ingredient to bring to anything that you wish to do well.

Centering is the ability to focus fully on your activity while at the same time being aware of your own inner presence. This enables you to gather your energy and channel it out into your activity. Don't let any thoughts about past or future interfere with how you feel in yourself here and now.

Your contact with the ground under your feet is significant because the energy of the earth inter-relates with your individual energy. This inter-exchange refreshes and stimulates us. When it is good a person is said to be 'grounded' and they will have stability, grace and confidence in their actions and movements. Your legs and feet are essential in this connection.

Hara is the centre of energy in man and woman (see page 12). Situated in the area of the abdomen, it is the natural point of balance physically, emotionally and spiritually and, as such, it is the focus when centering and grounding yourself.

The benefits to your Shiatsu

Being both grounded and centred in your hara is of vital importance when you give Shiatsu. There are many benefits:

- It adds depth to your treatment. As you begin to work more with your intuition, rather than with your intellect, you gain an instinctive touch and know just what is needed and where.
- You are able to move with a natural balance and control, using less muscle power.
- Your strength is given from your whole body, meaning that you become less tired and even feel refreshed and revitalised after giving a treatment.

How to centre

Centering and grounding exercises (see pages 133–136) can be practised regularly and in time you will be able to still your thoughts and come into your quiet self, by choice.

Before a Shiatsu treatment take a few minutes of meditation to gather yourself and centre in your hara.

Centering meditation

Sit in a way that is comfortable for you – in 'seisa' (see page 68), or cross legged or on a chair, with both feet flat on the ground. The important thing is to have a straight spine, which can be supported against a wall if necessary.

Close your eyes and sink inside yourself. Take a little time to atune to your inner world and become aware of any feelings or sensations that you have. Experience the weight of your body on the ground and its contact with the surface.

Breathe more deeply and on each out breath relax and let go of tensions in your body, especially in the shoulders and face. Allow your breathing to be natural and easy. Don't force it. Simply watch the breath come into your body and go out again. Visualise it flowing into you, filling your belly with warmth and light. Feel the muscles of your pelvis soften and open. As you breathe out imagine the energy from your hara streaming up your body, down your arms and out through your hands, which may begin to tingle and feel warm as they become energised. Stay like this for 5 to 10 minutes, or longer.

As you practise, centering yourself in this way becomes easier and need take only a few moments. However, it requires patience to allow your busy mind to subside. Each time your thoughts intrude simply bring your attention back to your breathing and concentrate on the feeling in your hara or hands.

Energising your hands

1 If you feel little awareness of your hands take some moments during the day simply to sit with them hanging down by your side. Relax your body and bring your attention to your hands. Don't think about your hands, rather actually experience the feeling sensation of being inside them. Initially it may be easier to practise this exercise using one hand only.

The action of gravity on your circulation will emphasise any feelings of warmth and tingling in your hands and you will gradually become aware of their aliveness.

2 Just before giving a treatment activate your hands by shaking them and rubbing the palms together. Your hands should feel warm and tingle when you stop.

The role of giver and receiver

Shiatsu is a sharing, and in the treatment both the giver and the receiver need to be open and relaxed and experience each moment of touch. In this way both are active and present to the Shiatsu and the process of healing. This experience can become like a meditation. The giver and the receiver each benefit and feel a deep fulfillment.

The giver

1 Your intent is all important

- Always approach a treatment with a feeling of respect and genuine care for your partner. However, maintain a certain detachment as you work. Your partner's condition and problems are not yours to take on.

- Do not give Shiatsu if you feel tired or upset in any way, as your condition will affect your partner and weaken your own energy.

- Keeping your attention on your partner and on your touch will give power to your treatment. Conversely, an absent mind and mechanical touch dilutes its potency.

2 Your own physical and psychological health is important

To give effective treatments you must be healthy. It is important for you to maintain and improve your own condition through diet and exercise (see page 109).

3 Talk to your partner

Your partner is in your hands during the treatment. Tell her what Shiatsu is and what to expect. Encourage her to give you feedback both during the treatment and afterwards. Discourage idle chatting when you work as this will only distract both of you.

It is important for you to know about any serious problems, illness or accidents that your partner has had. Question her about her health and any specific problems or pain presently troubling her.

The receiver

1 Be centred and aware

You will also benefit most fully from a Shiatsu treatment when you keep centred (see page 28) and focus on feeling the sensation of the touch. However, don't worry if at times your mind wanders or you fall asleep.

2 Be relaxed

Feel the total support of the ground as you lie down. Close your eyes and with each out breath let yourself soften and sink down. Trust in your partner and surrender to the treatment, allowing your body to be moved and manipulated without any help from you. Remember, you don't have to do anything except be there with awareness.

3 Give feedback

It helps your partner if you let her know what you are feeling. Don't suffer in silence if the pressure is too hard or too soft, or a stretch is uncomfortably painful. Share when a touch feels especially good.

Generally, though, keep talking to a minimum during the treatment. Afterwards much more can be said.

Approaching Shiatsu

Shiatsu is a living art whose form progresses as your practice develops. As you become increasingly able and comfortable in your Shiatsu, you will quite naturally use, adapt and create techniques to suit particular situations and the needs of your partner.

Very often the basic, simple Shiatsu techniques that you first learn are used again and again in preference to the more elaborate and complicated movements that are later acquired. For the essence of good Shiatsu is found in simplicity, and the quality that you bring to a treatment, rather than in complexity and style. Having said this, it is still important for you to be dextrous and skilled in technique. The number of different movements, manipulations and sequences that can be used is vast and you will come across many useful variations on the basic forms.

In this section a variety of techniques are described which work on the different areas of the body and show Shiatsu given to your partner in a variety of positions.

Practise and get to know the techniques; as you develop your Shiatsu treatment they will be there for you to select from and use in a way that suits the needs of your partner.

Learning to practise in parts

Initial contact

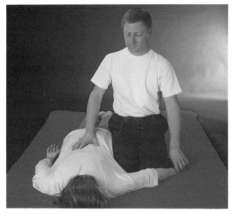 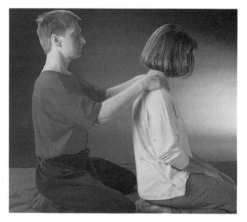

How you make contact with your partner is important. Let your touch be gentle. Allow some moments for your hands to rest on your partner before continuing with your treatment. A lot can happen in stillness and this first touch, when valued and not rushed, can allow both you and your partner time to relax and open up to each other. As your hands rest on him, take a few moments to centre yourself (see page 28).

Basic positions for the receiver

Shiatsu is most commonly given to your partner as she lies prone (face down) or supine (on her back).

Prone position

Ask your partner to lie on her stomach with her face turned to one side, arms by her side, palms uppermost and heels falling out. Encourage her to turn her head from time to time to avoid getting a stiff neck.

It is important that your partner is comfortable and can relax fully so make adjustments to her position to accommodate any stiffness she may have.

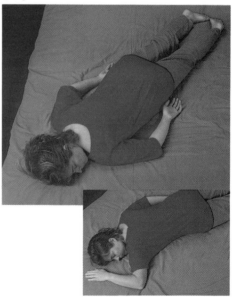

1 Tight shoulders and neck muscles can be eased by bending one or both arms and positioning them as shown.

STEP BY STEP GUIDE 33

2 A cushion can be placed under your partner's chest allowing more room for her head and relieving pressure on the neck.

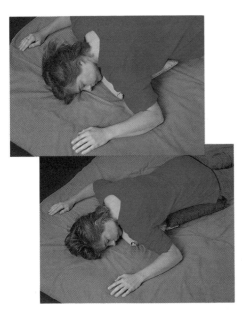

3 If your partner has a weak lower back, and feels any strain in that area with a cushion under her chest, place a second cushion under her belly to support the whole torso. Discomfort in her neck will now be eased without over arching and stressing the lower back.

   If your partner has persistent discomfort when lying in prone position, avoid using it. Instead work on the back area in supine, side or sitting positions.

Supine position

Ask your partner to lie on her back, arms relaxed by her side palms upper most with her legs slightly apart and feet falling out. Check that she is lying straight and make any adjustments to the

position that will increase her comfort and help relaxation.

1 If your partner has round shoulders or a curvature of the spine (kyphosis) she will often need a small cushion under her head.

2 Back pain can be eased by having the knees slightly bent and supported by a cushion.

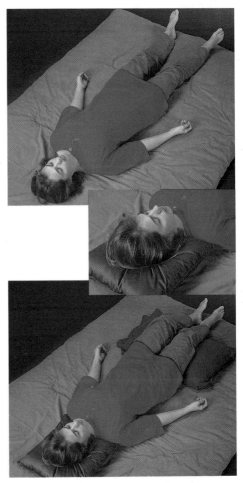

When your partner turns, advise her to move slowly and in her own time. Support and guide her as she moves into the new position. Straighten her arms, legs and head as necessary.

The back

Physical structure

The spine consists of 33 vertebrae. These bones fit together to form the spinal column and are attached to the skull and rib cage forming the main stay for the entire body, the axial skeleton. This is relatively rigid and supports the shoulders and pelvic girdle and the limbs. Layers of powerful muscle stabilise the many bones of the spine and strengthen the back. The spinal column also protects the spinal cord, the central nerve which extends out from the brain and down to the sacrum bone at the base of the spine. A huge number of nerves branch out from the brain and the spinal cord. These spread to all parts of the body and control the functioning and sensation of all the organs and systems.

Shiatsu technique

The strong muscles of the back mean that you can give deep Shiatsu to the area. Press more lightly on the lower back, however, as it is less protected.

Always have the utmost respect for a person's back. Work with care and without forcing especially if there are problems. Let the condition of the back 'lead' your treatment.

Prone position

1 Two hands

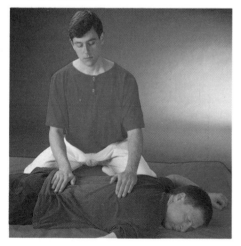

With your knees wide, sit comfortably on your heels, facing your partner. With one hand on his sacrum place the palm of the other flat between his shoulder blades. Pause, with relaxed shoulders. Then slowly begin to rock his hips. A good movement can develop as you allow your partner's own rhythm to emerge. (See page 24 for basic rocking technique.) Do this for a while then gently bring the rocking to a stop.

2 Side of hands

Face your partner's head and place the outside edges of your hands in the muscles along either side of the spine. In a rapid 'sawing' motion move up and down the length of the back with a firm pressure. (See page 20 for basic technique.)

This can also be done with one hand 'sawing' and your support hand resting on the sacrum.

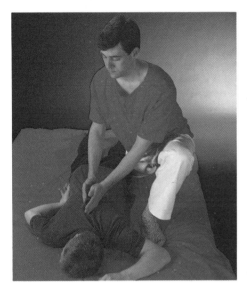

3 'Baby walking'

Come up onto all fours with your knees wide and palms on your partner's back. Relax your shoulders and back and let your belly drop.

Slowly walk with your hands all over his back shifting your weight forward as you move from hand to hand with a slightly circular motion. Be completely centred in your hara and allow your feeling and intuition to dictate where you place your hands. Linger on weaker areas that need more support.

Continue moving in this way until you feel your partner's body yield and become pliant. You can also include legs and arms as you 'baby walk' avoiding all joints and being sensitive to the lesser amounts of pressure these areas need. (See page 26 for basic 'baby walking' technique.)

4 Palming down the back

Place a support hand comfortably on the sacrum and use one hand to palm down the far side of the spine beginning between your partner's shoulder blades. Do this on the near side, adjusting your position to accommodate the different angle of your hands. Repeat if necessary.

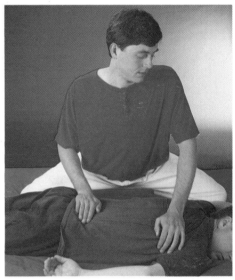

Palm pressure down each side of the spine in this way can effectively be given whilst gently rocking the sacrum with your support hand to encourage relaxation. (See page 20 for basic palming technique.)

5 Thumbs down back

Place your thumb pads on the muscles which run down each side of the spine where the inner branch of the Bladder channel is located, approximately two finger widths either side of the vertebrae. (See Channel chart, page 123.) Give perpendicular pressure to the body starting between the shoulder blades with your fingers fanning out over the ribs to stabilise and support you. As your partner exhales slowly bring your hips and weight forward to increase the

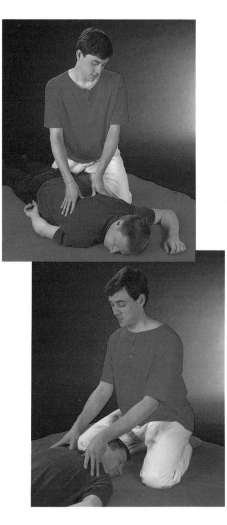

Now work in a similar way down the outer branch of the Bladder channel, situated approximately four finger widths out from the spine (see page 123).

The angle of the spine makes it easier to work on the upper back when you are at your partner's head. Begin at the top and press with both thumbs down the muscle each side of the spine to the mid back, as described above. Move your thumbs out and trace the outer branch of the Bladder channel working in a similar way. Repeat if necessary.

Stretches

1 Diagonal stretches

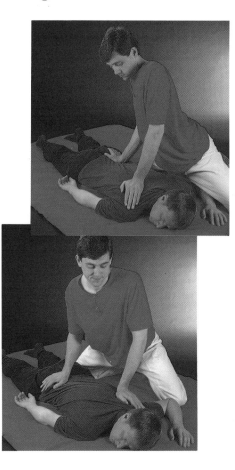

pressure given by your thumbs. Hold for some seconds, then quietly release by moving your weight back as he inhales. Work down your partner's back in this way, giving pressure at regular intervals, approximately one inch apart. Be easy and comfortable, with your elbows and hands firm, yet relaxed, and allow your movements to flow as you increase and release the pressure. Stay longer on the points that feel weak and low in energy. This stage can be repeated if necessary. (See page 18 for basic thumb technique.)

Kneel beside your partner with your knees apart and place one hand on his shoulder blade close to you and the other on the opposite hip. Anchor the heels of your hands on the bony parts with your fingers pointed in opposite directions. Face towards your partner's head and as you shift your weight forward to give pressure, let your hands move apart to stretch his back. Hold and repeat.

Then put your other hand on the other hip and shoulder blade and change your position to face towards your partner's feet. Lean forward and stretch as above. Hold and repeat.

2 Spine stretch

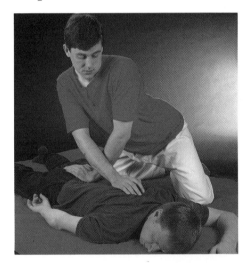

Face your partner, cross your arms and place one hand securely on his sacrum bone with your fingers pointing towards the feet. Place your other hand on the spine of his upper back with your fingers pointing towards his head. Bring your weight forward and stretch the spine by moving your hands apart. Hold and repeat.

Now, keeping the pressure of your sacrum hand constant, move your other hand down your partner's spine at regular intervals, each time leaning in and stretching.

3 Sacrum stretch

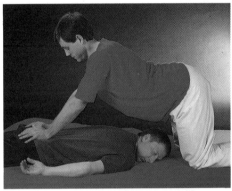

Have your knees above your partner's head. Lean forward and place your palms over her sacrum with the heels catching the tilt of the pelvic bone. Lean your weight through your hands giving strong pressure in a forward direction as well as down. Hold in a relaxed way for some time.

Supine position

The back can be effectively treated when your partner lies in supine position by slipping your hands under the body and letting its weight sink into your hands.

Also various ways of stretching and twisting can be used to release and relax the back muscles.

1 Fingers in the back muscles

Stand astride your partner. Lift one side of his chest as you slide your free hand under his upper back, as high up as possible. Ease your other hand under the opposite side so that both palms lie flat against the back muscles, finger tips opposite each other on either side of the spine.

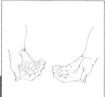

Position of hands under back

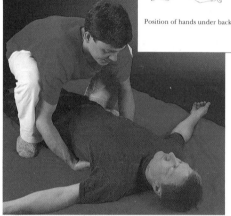

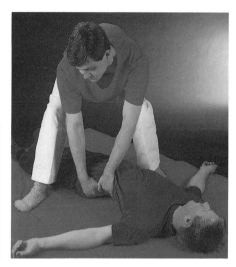

Stroke rhythmically in this way down to his hips, then slide your hands right under his buttocks. Raise one side and gently bounce.

Repeat the sequence down his other side.

2 Twist with one leg

Bend your partner's leg up and guide his knee over the other straight leg, pushing it down and away from you. At the same time secure his diagonally opposite shoulder to create a spinal twist as

Support your knuckles on the ground and bend your fingers up and into the muscle. Hold, letting the body weight of your partner sink into your finger tips. Release and move down either side of the spine, giving pressure in this way at regular intervals.

Use the flat of your finger tips over the kidney area and lumbar vertebrae down to the sacrum.

Stretches

1 Side lift

Face your partner's head as you stand with your legs on either side of his torso. Work on one side at a time using both of your hands alternately to lift the torso as your hands slide up and over his side.

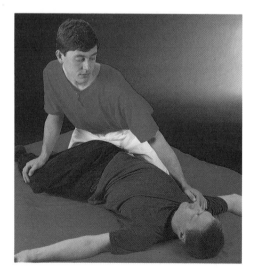

you stretch your two hands apart.
Slowly release and repeat on the
other side.

3 Twist with both legs

Bend your partner's legs up and
guide both knees over to one side.
Secure the diagonally opposite
shoulder as you hold his knees
down to give a stretch. Do not force
past the point of resistance.
Hold and release slowly and
repeat on the other side.

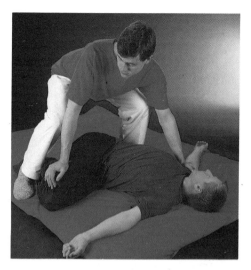

Hips and buttocks

Physical structure

The two hip bones are joined by the sacrum to form the bowl-shaped
pelvic girdle. This supports and connects the upper body with the legs,
with its sturdy form distributing the body's weight from the lumbar
vertebrae evenly through the sacrum and hip joints into the legs and feet.
It is these important joints that give flexibility and mobility to the whole
body and allow the pelvis to accommodate a large variety of movements.
The pelvic structure also acts as a shock absorber which protects the spine
and upper body from the impact of jarring motion.

In addition, the pelvic bowl contains and protects a complex of systems
in the abdomen – digestive, urinatory and reproductive – as well as a
mass of muscles, ligaments, veins and arteries, nerves, lymphs nodes and
so on.

Shiatsu technique

Good and deep Shiatsu, including stretches, movement and rotations of
the joints and legs, will stimulate the pelvic area and benefit the whole
body.

Prone position

1 Thumb pressure on sacrum

Explore the area of the sacrum.
Feel for the outline of the
triangular shaped bone and use
your fingers to press over it,
seeking out the four pairs of
indentations (see illustration).
Press each pair with your thumbs,
working down towards the coccyx.
The top two pairs are larger and
easier to find than the lower ones.
Pressing in the hollows will

stimulate the nerves and feel good, so ask your partner for feedback. Work slowly and thoroughly.

Place your hand over the one side of the sacrum and use the thumb of your other hand to press along the opposite side of the bone, lingering on tender places. Work like this along the other edge of the bone.

the muscles to loosen any tension.

Rest one hand on her sacrum/ buttock and use your elbow to work in to the muscle of the far side buttock.

Repeat this on the other side.

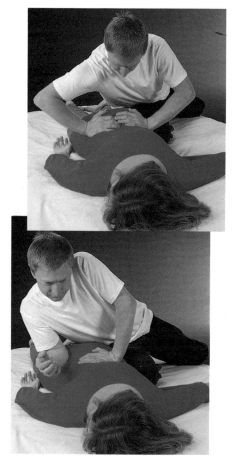

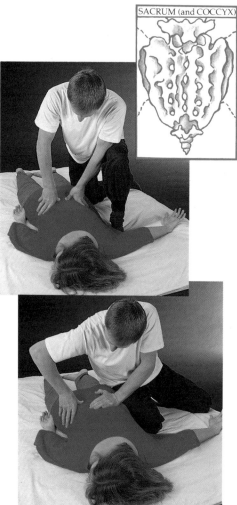

2 Hip squeeze

Use the heels of your hands to squeeze her hips together, rotating

Supine position

In this position the hip joints can be rotated and stretched to encourage flexibility and prevent energy stagnation in the pelvis, lower back and legs.

1 Rotation and stretch – one leg

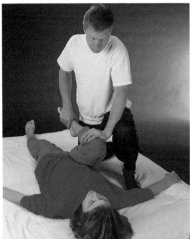

stretch. Rotate a few times in one direction and then in the other.

As your confidence and skill improves with practice use only one hand to support and rotate your partner's leg. Place your other hand on her hara and 'listen' with it. When you feel any tightness in her hips as you rotate, press into her hara more firmly.

Support the back of her knee as you slowly straighten the leg, and then work on the other in a similar way.

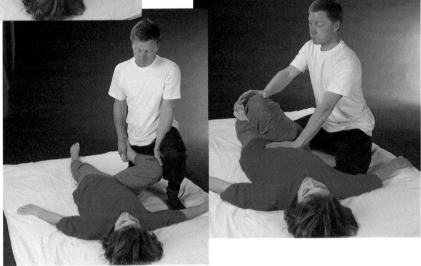

Kneel with one leg up. Face your partner's head and bend the leg close to you with one hand guiding her knee and the other supporting her foot. Press her knee to her chest as you move your weight forward onto your foot. Gradually increase the stretch to its comfortable limit and hold.

Release a little, then gently rotate the knee. Feel for tight spots in the hip as you circulate. Linger on these. Encourage your partner to breathe deeply and relax into the

2 Rotation and stretch – both legs

Standing astride your partner, lift both her legs and press the knees gently to her chest. Keep your shoulders relaxed and your own knees slightly bent as you lean your weight forward. Hold without forcing and then release slightly. Open her knees and press them again to her chest so that they fall to each side of her body.

Now slowly rotate both legs holding the knees together in wide circulations. Repeat, circulating in the other direction.

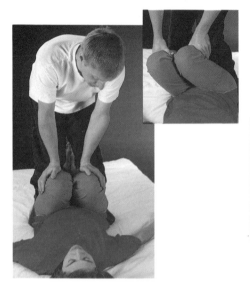

3 Hip roll and bounce

Pick up her hips by sliding your hands under each side of her body and roll them from hand to hand.

Then gently bounce her pelvis up and down, supporting it firmly between both of your hands.

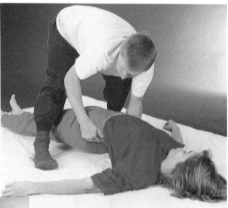

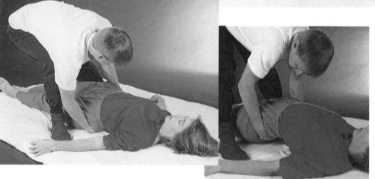

The abdomen

Physical structure

The abdomen is the extremely soft and delicate belly area which contains the vital organs of digestion and assimilation and of the urinary and reproductive systems. In women the womb is important as the centre of creation. The abdomen is largely unprotected by skeletal structure. While it is supported and contained by the pelvic bowl, with the diaphragm and ribs defining the upper part and the spinal column bracing the back, the whole front area relies only on layers of muscle to uphold and secure its position and form.

Hara

The hara is situated in the abdomen, being centred in the lower belly beneath the navel. It is not a physical organ in the body but an area which must be understood 'energetically' as the seat of life, strength and power of a person (see page 12).

The condition of the hara, as reflected in the abdomen, should be firm and yielding with strong yet relaxed muscle tone. In good health the area beneath the navel will feel sturdy and full yet pliant. It should protrude slightly more than the upper part.

Shiatsu to the hara

In Japan Shiatsu given to the hara is considered to be the most important and fundamental aspect of a treatment. In fact there are specialists who train exclusively to work on the hara and this very ancient therapy is known as 'Ampuku'. A skilled Ampuku therapist can diagnose and cure sickness by working only on the hara.

A great deal of practice and experience is needed to develop the sensitivity which enables accurate diagnosis of the hara and the profound use of Shiatsu upon it. However, hara Shiatsu can be given even by a beginner and be an important and valuable part of a treatment. Penetrating pressure used with awareness will stimulate the intestines, bladder and reproductive organs and encourage the release of toxins, congestion and tensions.

Sensitive work given to the hara is very relaxing and extremely beneficial to a person's overall well being.

Shiatsu technique

Many people are not used to having their belly touched, so always make contact slowly and gently. Rest your hand on their hara for a time before giving pressure.

Always position yourself close to your partner at hip level and keep your hara open and turned towards her. Be centred as you work slowly, gently and deeply with your full attention. Your touch needs to be supportive to allow your partner to relax.

Supine position

1 Holding

Sit beside your partner and place one hand on her hara with your other hand resting on your knee. Relax your shoulders and centre yourself in your hara as you breathe fully and naturally, harmonising your breath with your partner's. Stay like this for some time and allow your own sensitivity to tune in to your partner's physical and mental presence.

A variation is to face your partner and slide one hand under the small of her back, palm uppermost. Rest your other palm

on her belly, 'sandwiching' her
hara. Hold in a relaxed way with
awareness of your partner and of
your breathing.

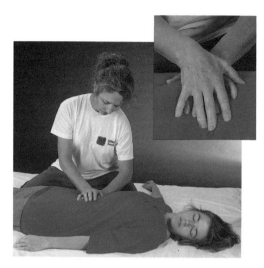

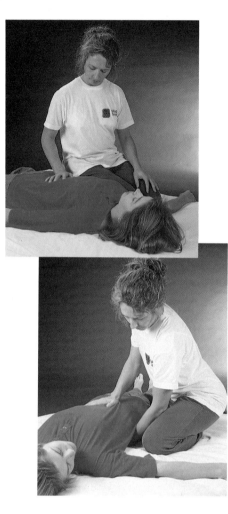

heels as you pull back with your
fingers. Let a rhythm of movement
develop as your hands work in
unison supporting each other
creating a wave like motion over
the hara. Keep your hands and
shoulders relaxed as you work over
the area of the abdomen
thoroughly.

3 Pressing around the hara

Face your partner and place your
'support' hand over her navel. Use
the side of your active hand to
press into the hara as she exhales.
Begin at the top and move around

2 Wave movement

Face your partner and place one
hand over her navel with the heel
resting on the near side muscles,
fingers pointing away. Place your
other hand on top of the first hand
with the finger tips extending past
the fingers of the underhand.

Use the heel of your hands to
push the muscles of the abdomen
away from you. Then raise the

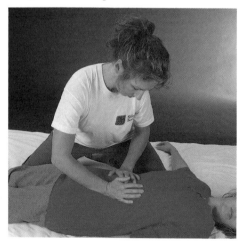

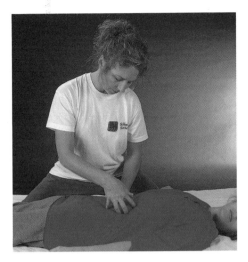

the far side to the centre bottom. Change your support hand and continue pressing around and up the near side to the top. Work in the same direction as the flow of the colon.

Repeat the circulation using the tips of all your fingers to give gradual and deep pressure. Be sensitive to areas of tenderness and pain. Do not force or work fast.

Legs

Physical structure

The legs and feet are designed primarily to support and transport us. They are attached to the hip bones by a sturdy joint and large muscles. Major nerves which activate the legs pass from the lumbar vertebrae and sacrum through the pelvis, into the thighs and down the legs to the feet.

Knees and ankles

Both the knee and ankle joints are weight bearing and therefore susceptible to physical stress and damage. The knee joints are intricate and designed to provide flexibility of movement whilst both supporting the weight of, and balancing, the whole body. They are especially vulnerable to injury when they are braced and held tense.

Shiatsu technique

In general, leg and foot Shiatsu can be firm and deep. Take care when you work around the lower legs and ankles as this area is painful in some people.

When the Shiatsu technique is being described on one leg, always work on the other leg in the same way, to balance the person, unless there is a reason not to.

Warning

Do not press around the ankles and lower leg during pregnancy. Pressure here can encourage miscarriage. If necessary give palm healing or a very light touch only.

Prone position

1 Palm and thumb pressure – leg straight

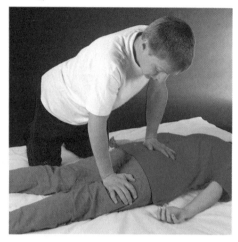

Kneel facing your partner and maintain even pressure with your support hand on her sacrum. Palm down each leg with your other hand (see page 20 for basic technique). Avoid the back of the knee and work more lightly on the calf muscles. Squeeze her ankle.

2 Thumbs in back of knee

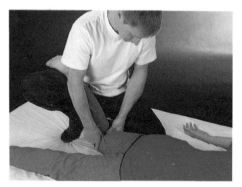

With your partner's leg bent and resting on your thigh, use both of your thumbs to press gently into the soft area at the back of her knee.

3 Side of the leg

Bend your partner's leg out to the side as shown. Support both her knee and ankle as you do this. Rest your support hand on her hip and palm and thumb down the exposed side of the leg. Use lighter pressure on the lower part and brush off her foot.

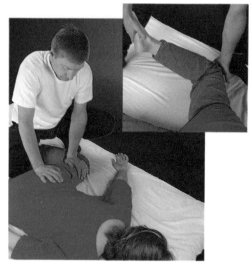

Stretches

1 One leg bend

Kneel facing your partner, rest one hand on her lower back and bend her leg up close to you. Support the ankle and gently press the heel towards her buttocks. Hold at the maximum stretch then release halfway and repeat, stretching the foot towards the opposite buttock. Release halfway and repeat again, stretching the foot towards the outside of her hip. Hold and release.

2 Achilles tendon stretch

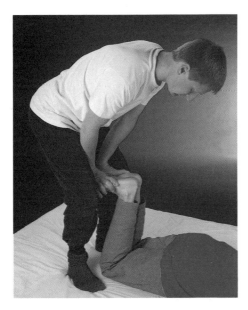

Bend both legs up so that the lower legs are perpendicular to the floor. Press down on the ball of both feet with your hands, stretching the back of the ankles and the achilles tendons. Hold, then release and gently straighten the legs.

Supine position

The leg joints have an increased opportunity for movement when your partner lies on her back, usually giving you greater access to the tsubos and channels.

1 Palm and thumb pressure – leg straight

Kneel facing your partner, with your support hand on her hara (below the navel). Use the palm of your active hand to give firm pressure along the thigh.

Roll and knead the thigh muscle first if it is hard and tight, that is, jitsu.

Move your position so that you can stretch your partner's foot with your hand and use your thumb to give lighter pressure on the lower

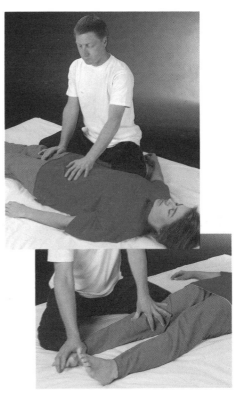

leg. Press the muscles running along the outside edge of the leg bone.

To 'lift' this muscle, increase the stretch on the foot. Work down the leg 2 or 3 times.

2 Side of leg

Bend your partner's leg up with her foot flat on the ground. Hold her knee and rest your other hand on her hara. Give pressure along the outside of the leg by pulling it onto your knee. Keep well balanced with relaxed shoulders and work slowly and deeply along the thigh. Press more gently on the lower leg.

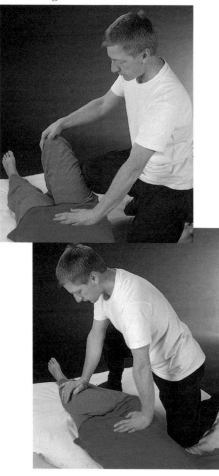

Stretch your partner's thigh by pushing her knee away from you. Hold and use your other hand to palm down the taut side muscles of her thigh.

3 Knee joint

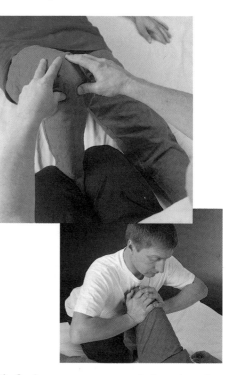

Sit facing your partner's head and secure her foot between your knees. Use your thumbs to press around the knee cap. Feel for the soft areas. Also sink your fingers into the back of her knee and hold.

Now, with the heels of your hands, vigorously rub the muscles around the knee at the side and up into the thigh.

4 Inside leg

Bend your partner's leg out to the side and place the sole of her foot against her other leg by the knee. Stretch it by pressing the knee down. Then support it on your thigh as you rest your support hand on her hara and palm slowly down the inside of her leg. Use the heel of your hand, with a deeper pressure on the larger thigh muscles.

Now use your thumb to press down the leg.

Reposition your partner's foot and place it against her ankle and then against her inner thigh. This will expose facets of her leg and different channels to work on. Repeat the process of giving pressure in each of these positions.

Stretches

Straight leg stretch

Stand at your partner's feet, pick up one foot and hold it in both hands. Lean back and stretch her leg, shaking it slightly as you pull.

Alternatively both legs can be stretched simultaneously. Support the heels in your hands and rest your forearms on your thighs as you lean back and pull.

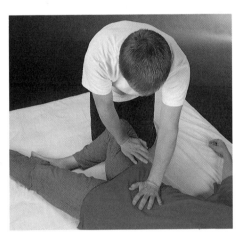

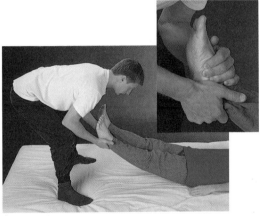

Hip rotations (see pages 40–42) also serve to stretch the legs. They form a good transition movement between different leg positions.

Feet

Physical structure

The intricate structure of each foot involves 26 small bones which form an arch and operate together as a fluid whole. This is necessary so that the feet can balance on and mould to uneven surfaces and absorb much of the shock caused when they strike the ground as we walk, run or jump. All of the toes are needed for balance.

Shiatsu technique

When Shiatsu technique is described for one foot always work on the other foot in the same way to balance the person, unless there is a reason not to.

WARNING:

Do **not** press around the ankles during pregnancy.

Prone position

1 Elbow and thumb pressure

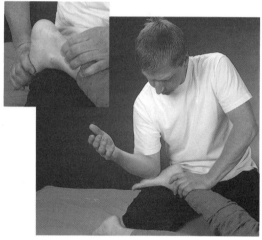

Sit back on your heels with wide knees and support your partner's lower leg and foot across your thigh. Vary the angle of your elbow as you use it to give Shiatsu to the sole of her foot. Rest your support hand comfortably on her leg.

Then, supporting her foot with your hand, use the thumb of your other hand to press over the sole. Squeeze the ankle along each side of the achilles tendon, around the edge of the foot and down the toes. (See supine position, All over treatment.)

2 Kidney palm healing

Bend your partner's leg and support it on your thigh. Use your thumb in the sole of her foot over kd 1 (see illustration) and give firm pressure. Simultaneously, place your support hand over the kidney area on her back, on the same side, and hold for some time. Try to sense for a connecting link between your two hands. You can further stimulate kd 1 by slightly rotating the skin over the tsubo as you press.

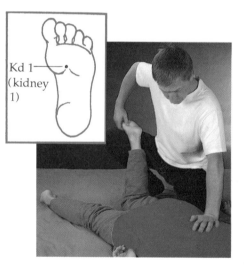

Kd 1 (kidney 1)

3 Toe pull

Standing, bend your partner's leg and support it with a hand under the instep. Begin with the big toe and pinch along its length. Lift the leg slightly letting the toe bear the whole weight. Shake slightly and release. Repeat this process pulling and shaking all the toes.

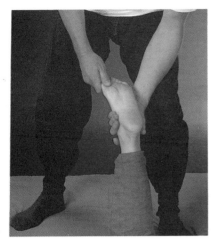

Supine position

1 All over treatment

Position yourself in such a way that it feels easy to use your thumb or middle finger knuckle, to press into the bottom of your partner's foot. Give pressure all over the sole and heel, lingering on the tender spots. Pinch the achilles tendon and around the outside edge of the heel and foot. Squeeze the toes, rotate and pull them.

2 Top of foot

Support your partner's foot in your hand while using your thumb to press between the bones on the top of the foot.

Press around the ankle joint, seeking out the soft and tender points between the bones.

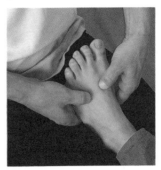

Stretches

1 Ankle joint – rotate, stretch and flex

Rest your partner's leg over your thighs and clasp and support the top of the ankle just above the joint. Hold the foot with your other

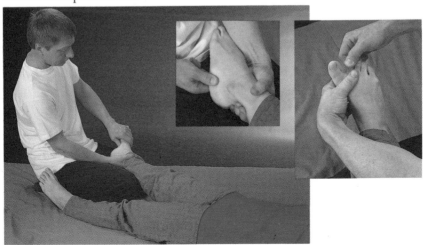

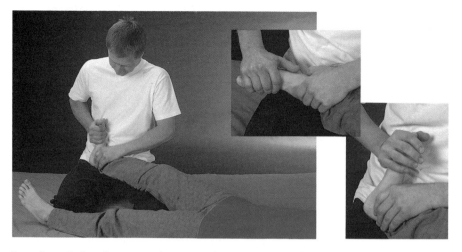

hand and slowly rotate it around, first in one direction and then in the other. Keep the foot close to your hara and emphasise the rotation with the movement of your upper body.

Then stretch the foot forward with your hand, leaning your weight into the stretch. Hold.

Next, flex the foot. Again, lean your weight into the stretch and hold.

Arms and hands

Physical structure

The arms and hands are a complex assemblage of bones and joints held in place by tendons and muscles. They are attached to the highly mobile shoulder joints and thus they have a wide range of movement suitable for everyday activity and survival. The hands have evolved into a structure of unique dexterity with the thumb and fingers being able to act like pincers.

Shiatsu technique

When the Shiatsu technique is described for one arm, always work on the other arm in the same way to balance the person, unless there is a reason not to, for example, injury to that arm.

Prone position

1 Loosening the arm

With your partner's palm turned upwards, rest your support hand on her upper back, sliding your other hand under her shoulder joint. Lift and shake the shoulder joint with small, rapid loosening movements. Continue in this manner down her arm to her hand. Repeat if necessary.

Then support her shoulder, and, firmly and quickly, roll the muscles of her arm. Avoid the elbow joint. Repeat if necessary.

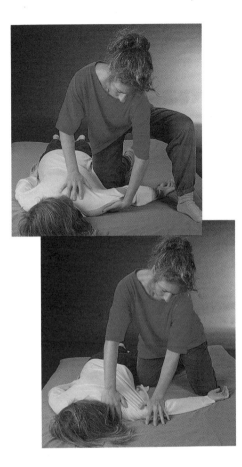

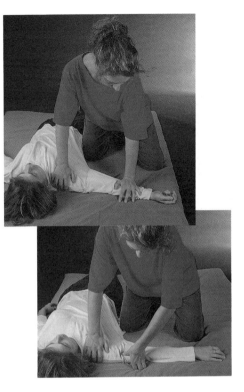

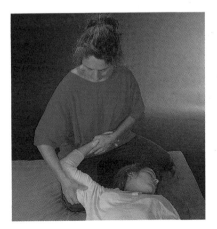

Supine position

1 Arm out to the side

Lay your partner's arm out to the side, palm uppermost. Rest your support hand on her shoulder and press slowly down the inside of the arm. Avoid the elbow joint and work down to the hand. Press down on her palm and hold. You can repeat, using your thumb to trace the channels.

Turn your partner's hand and place the palm face down. Keep your support hand on her shoulder and palm down the exposed area of the arm. You can repeat, using your thumb to press along the channels.

2 Arm above the head

Sit by your partner's head with her arm stretched up and resting across your thighs. Elbow bent, hold the back of her hand to your hara and work along the arm squeezing it between your thumb and fingers from the armpit to the hand.

3 Arm across the chest

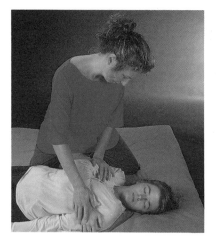

Take your partner's arm across her chest and secure it with one hand as you apply palm or thumb pressure along the exposed side, from her shoulder.

Stretches

1 Overhead stretch

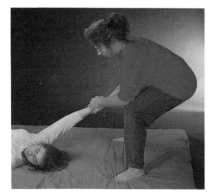

One arm – stand behind your partner's head, stretch back one arm and hold it firmly at the wrist. Pull it, leaning back to increase the stretch over her head. Bend your knees and keep your hands low, to ensure that the stretch pulls horizontally and not just upwards. Hold and release and place the arm back to the side.

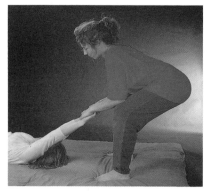

Both arms – take both arms over your partner's head and hold securely by the wrists. Slowly squat down as you lean back resting your elbows on your knees. Hold the stretch then release slowly.

2 Wrist stretches

Sit beside your partner and bend her arm, keeping the elbow on the

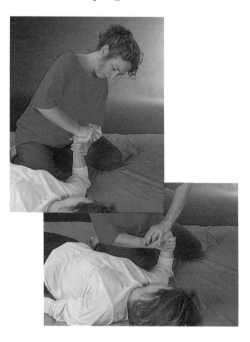

ground. Support the underside of her wrist firmly with one hand and use the other hand to bend it gently, pressing the hand forward and over. Hold the stretch, then bend the wrist backwards in the opposite direction and again hold and release.

Hands

1 Palm stretch

Hold your partner's hand in both of your hands, palm uppermost, and lace your little fingers under her three middle fingers. Stretch her palm with your thumbs, by drawing them across and out to the sides. Press around the whole area of the palm with your thumbs.

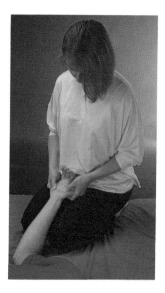

2 Finger pull

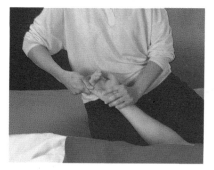

Beginning with the thumb, rotate, squeeze and pull along the length of each finger in turn. Make sure you work right up to the fingertips and off the ends.

3 Back of hand

Use your thumbs to press along the back of the hand between the bones.

Squeeze the soft fleshy part between the thumb and first finger and hold. This is an important tsubo (L4) for waste elimination and general toning up of the body and it may be tender.

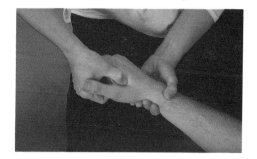

Chest

Physical structure

The chest is formed from 12 paired ribs which encircle and protect the very delicate lungs and heart. They are attached to the 12 thoracic vertebrae at the back and joined at the front by the sternum or breast bone. The diaphragm muscle separates the abdomen from the chest cavity which is sealed and airtight. The movement of the diaphragm and the muscles of the rib cage cause the volume of space inside the lungs to increase and decrease and in this way breathing takes place.

Shiatsu technique

Work with gentleness on the chest as many people will feel sensitive and vulnerable and may be apprehensive of your touch.

Very often the front of a person's body will be relatively weak (kyo) so use steady, gradually deepening pressure to tonify the area. This will help to release tension in the back and shoulders.

Supine position

1 Pressing along the top of the chest

2 Pressing up the breastbone

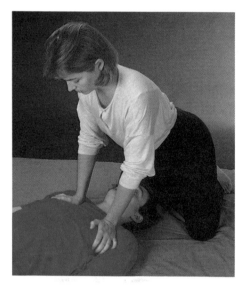

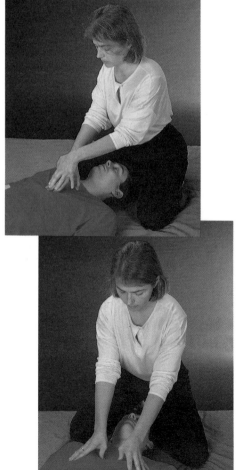

Kneel behind your partner's head and place the heels of your hands together on the centre of the upper chest beneath the collar bone, with fingers pointing out to the side. Lean your weight forward keeping your arms firm and give steady pressure. Hold, release and move your hands apart. Move along the muscle out to the shoulders, giving pressure at regular intervals.

Place the three middle fingers of the hand on the bottom of your partner's breast bone, with the corresponding fingers of your other hand resting on top. Press down and hold. Let the fingers of the under hand be passive and the fingers of the top hand give the pressure. Release and move about one inch up the breast bone. Again press and hold. Proceed in this way slowly up the centre of the chest to the collar bone.

Now use your thumbs and press each side of the breast bone in the notches between the ribs. Begin at the bottom and work slowly up to the collar bone. Press lightly at first and increase the pressure as your partner opens to your touch.

The shoulders

Physical structure

The shoulders work with the neck to provide a firm structure on which to support the head. Their extensive mobility comes about largely because the shoulder girdle is floating, having the collar bones as its only point of attachment to the main supportive structure, the axial skeleton. The collar bones connect to the top of the breast bone in the front of the chest, with layers of muscles alone fastening and stabilising the shoulder blades to the axial skeleton at the back.

Shiatsu technique

The whole body can benefit from sensitive penetrating Shiatsu given thoroughly to the entire shoulder region.

Prone position

1 Loosening the shoulders

Stand astride your partner, his arms away from his side. Slide your hands under his shoulders. Lift and shake each shoulder alternately with small rapid movements. As you do this, move your hands along the muscles from the shoulder joints to his neck. His head should remain on the ground without straining the neck.

With the flat of your fingers fully wrapped over his shoulders, lean back to exert pressure on the muscles. Move each hand alternately, working between the shoulder joints and neck.

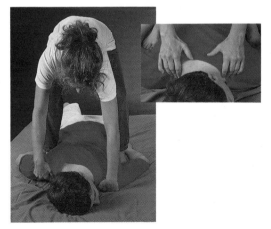

2 The shoulder blade

the point up to the shoulder. Seek out areas that feel good to touch. Cover the whole area thoroughly.

Supine position

1 Pressing down on the shoulders

Kneel behind your partner's head and cup his shoulders with your fingers curling over the top of the joints. Keep your arms straight as you lean your weight forward, pinning down his shoulders. Hold and release.

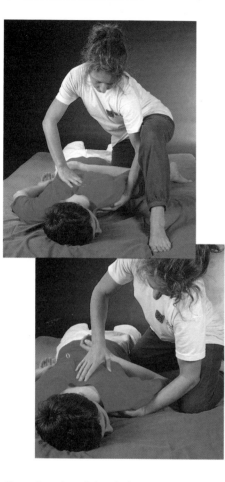

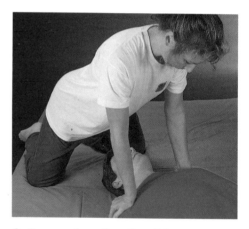

2 Loosening the shoulders

Cup the shoulder joint as you gently bend your partner's arm behind his back. Be sensitive to his flexibility and, if necessary, support his arm on your knee. Shake his shoulder up and down to loosen it and expose the movement of the shoulder blade.

Work the tsubos around the blade. Let your fingers or thumbs sink in and slide under the bone as the muscles relax. To give yourself more support and leverage, work with one leg up.

Keep his shoulder cupped and give pressure with your thumb diagonally across the blade from

Kneel beside your partner and stretch his arm over his chest. Slide your free hand under the slightly raised shoulder, then straighten his arm by his side again. Slip your hand under his upper back on the other side of his arm and with the fingers of both hands work around his shoulder blade. Let the weight of his body provide a deep and passive pressure as you curl your fingers into the muscle. Work around the shoulder blade along the top of his shoulder, squeezing and kneading the muscle. (See opposite.) Work on the other side in a similar way.

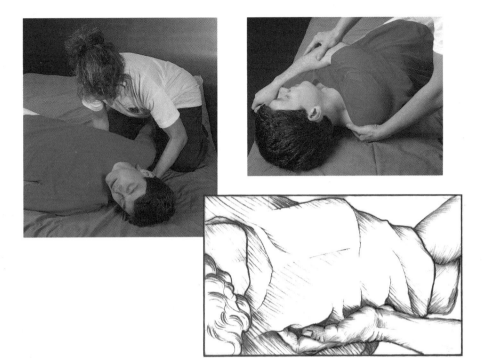

The neck

Physical structure

The neck connects the head with the rest of the body. Its slender form contains the voice box, vertebrae protecting the spinal cord, passages for food and air, major blood vessels, nerves and channels. An intricate system of muscles supports the neck and this allows it a very comprehensive range of movement.

Shiatsu technique

Keeping the neck flexible and in good condition is important. Regular Shiatsu will help ensure that tensions do not become permanent and create serious problems. The muscles of the back and side of the neck will often hold tension and be tender, especially where they meet the rim of the skull. To give good Shiatsu to the neck requires practice, time and sensitivity.

Prone position

Work on the neck is not easy in this position. You can simply draw your hands from your partner's shoulders up the neck and off her head.

Supine position

Sit comfortably above your partner's head.

1 Checking the neck

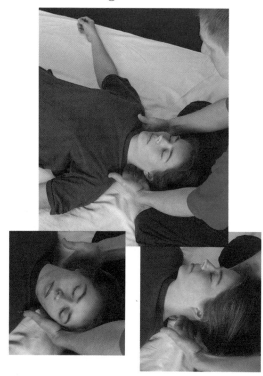

Lightly use the tips of your fingers to press the muscles on either side of your partner's neck and along the cervical vertebrae, to give you an idea of the condition of the neck. Feel for lumps, tight muscles and misaligned vertebrae. Support the head and gently roll it to each side. Notice the flexibility and degree of relaxation of the muscles.

2 Working on each side of the neck

Place your hands at each side of your partner's head with your fingers curling around the back of her skull and your thumbs lying in front of the ears. Turn her head to one side, support it with one hand and press into the muscles on the underside of the neck with the fingers of your other hand. Let the

weight of your partner's head increase the strength of pressure you give. You can also move your fingertips in small circles on her neck moving the skin over the muscles as you press.

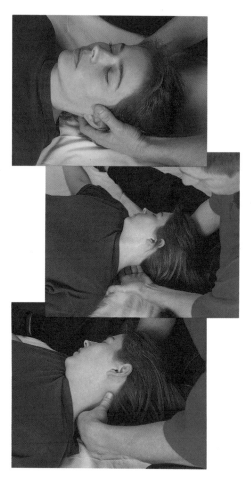

Now work along the muscle just below the rim of the skull with your thumb. Begin at the side and work towards the centre, pressing into the muscle and up under the skull. Give gentle pressure that gradually increases and penetrates whilst still being comfortable to your partner. To increase pressure, roll her head towards your thumb pad. Move slowly and with care, holding points that are tender to touch.

Gently turn her head and work in the same way on the other side of the neck.

Neck stretches

1 Side stretch

Slide one hand under your partner's neck at the base of the skull and place your other hand over her shoulder joint. Push the shoulder away as you slightly lift and move her head towards her other shoulder. Don't turn her head. Hold the stretch and release it slowly.

Then, turn your partner's head to one side, and support her cheek on your hand with your thumb and first finger around her ear. Now move her face towards her shoulder; cup her other shoulder simultaneously and press it away to stretch the neck. Hold and release. Repeat both stretches on the other side.

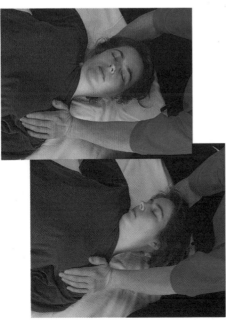

2 Forward stretch

Support the back of your partner's neck and head with both hands. Lift it slowly by coming up onto your knees. Move your position forward as you stretch the back of her neck, tucking her chin into her chest. Hold the stretch at the point of resistance and ask your partner to breathe more deeply and to relax fully on her out breath.

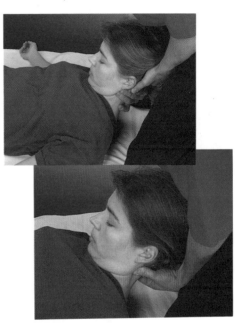

Now release the stretch slowly, supporting the back of your partner's neck and head. As the neck straightens squeeze it between your thumb and fingers. Keep her chin tucked in as you do this to stretch the back of the neck slightly. Release and gently lay her head back on the ground.

Head and face

Physical structure

That remarkable and extremely complex organ, the brain, is completely surrounded and protected by the skull with only the eyes, the windows of the soul, being exposed to the world. Irregular and angular bones fit together at the front of the skull to form the structure of the face. This is covered with very fine and delicate muscles which create the wealth of facial expressions we use. The entire head is supported by 7 vertebrae in the neck.

Shiatsu technique

1 Kneading the scalp

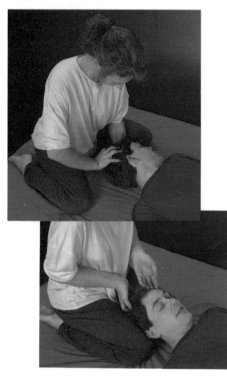

Turn your partner's head, support it in one hand and use the fingers and thumb pads of your other hand to knead and massage firmly over the exposed surface of his scalp. Move the skin over the skull bones in a way that feels good. Remember to include the hair line.

Then support his head in your other hand and massage the other side.

Rest your partner's head between your knees and run the backs of your finger nails slowly through his hair beginning just before the hair line. Work from the centre, out to both sides and back again.

2 Relaxing the face

Smooth across the skin on your partner's face with your finger and thumb tips, working out from the centre line and upwards. Follow the bone formation with your hands working in unison, mirroring each other's movements.

Squeeze his eye brows between your thumbs and first fingers beginning from the inside edge

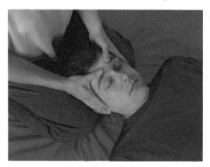

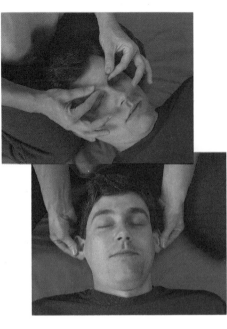

around the edge of his ears pinching and pulling them outwards.

3 Pressing tsubos

Use your finger and thumb tips to press the tsubos of his head and face. Work slowly and gently.

and work out. Finish by firmly smoothing over them.

Squeeze both ear lobes, pull them down and hold. Then work

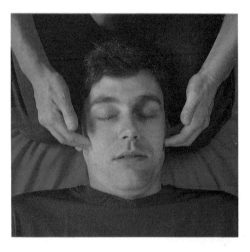

Side Shiatsu

For people who cannot comfortably lie prone, for example during pregnancy, or for those who are unable to turn the head easily, side Shiatsu is good. It is also a useful position to use when working on shoulder tension.

Position

Lie your partner on her side and support her head with a cushion. Bend her top leg and keep her underleg straight. You can also place a cushion under the bent knee if necessary. Pull her under arm to straighten her shoulders and to stop her falling forwards. Balance her upper arm across the top of her body.

Shiatsu technique

Work fully on one side and then help your partner to turn over and repeat your sequence of techniques on her other side. Sit back between your heels (in seisa, see page 68) close to your partner's upper back and support her with your body as you give Shiatsu to her head, neck and shoulders.

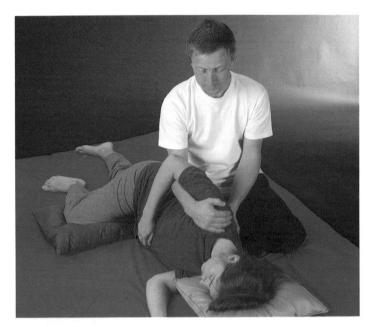

*Position for
giving Side Shiatsu*

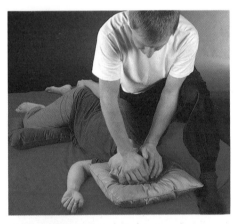

1 Head press

Come up on your knees, slowly
lean your weight forward and
press down gently with both hands
on the side of your partner's head.
Hold.

Change your hand position and
press again. Hold, then release.

Now include the jaw and the side
of the face in this. Press with care
and only in a way that feels
comfortable and safe to your
partner.

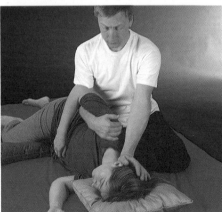

2 Neck and shoulder stretch

Slide your arm under your
partner's arm and curve your hand
up and over her shoulder. Place
the heel of your other hand under
the rim of her skull and gently
push it away as you pull on the
shoulder.

If you need more balance, bend
one leg up or have it out straight as
you work. Hold the stretch and
release.

3 Pressing into the neck

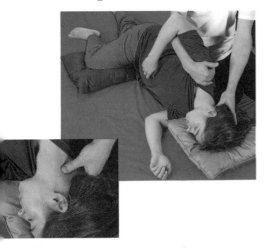

Keep your arm supporting your partner's shoulder and use the thumb of your hand to press under the rim of the skull. Begin behind her ear and work slowly along towards the spine. As you do this, slightly pull on her shoulder to stretch her neck as you give pressure.

Now press down the neck, squeezing it between your thumb and fingers. Again gently pull on the shoulder as you do this.

4 Shoulder pressure

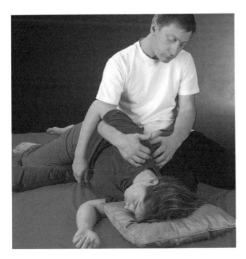

Still supporting your partner's shoulder use the fingers of both your hands to press down along the muscle of the top of her shoulders. Begin at the base of her neck and work along to the shoulder joints. Lean your weight back to increase the pressure.

5 Loosening the shoulder blades

Push your partner's shoulder back slightly to release her shoulder blade. Press the muscle around and under her shoulder blade with your fingers. Work the area thoroughly. Now support the shoulder joint firmly with one hand, curl your fingers under the edge of her shoulder blade and 'lift' it. Hold and release.

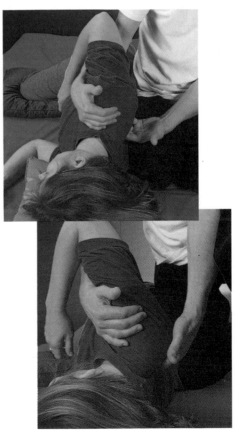

6 Arm rotation and stretch

Come up on your knees and cup the top of your partner's shoulder joint firmly in one hand. Support her arm with your other hand by holding it at the wrist.

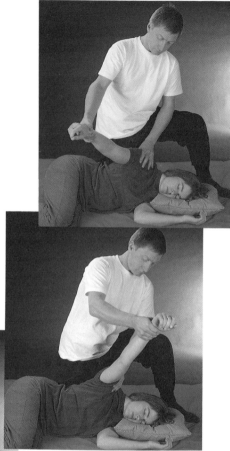

Slowly rotate her arm, keeping it straight as you move it out to the front, up and around to the back and so on. Echo the rotation of the arm with the movement of your body. Rotate 2 or 3 times.

Now clasp your partner's wrist with both hands and stretch it upwards and slightly back. Hold and release.

Always rotate and stretch the arm carefully and comfortably within the range of flexibility of your partner.

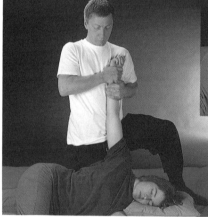

7 Rubbing and pressing the back

Sit close to your partner's hips and place one hand over her chest. Use the palm and heel of your other hand to rub over her back and shoulders. Use the 2 fingers on the same hand to rub firmly up and down either side of the spine.

Give thumb pressure down the muscles on either side of the spine.

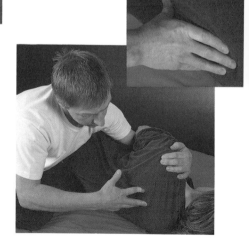

8 Spinal twist

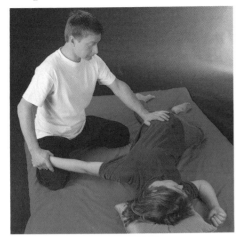

Kneel and face your partner. Secure her arm as you place one hand on her hip and push it away. Ask your partner to breathe more deeply and relax into the stretch. Hold it and release slowly. Caution: do this with sensitivity and care.

9 Holding the hara

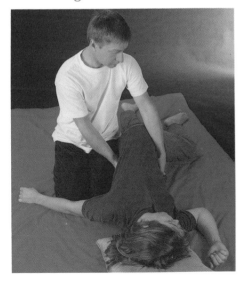

Sit beside your partner and sandwich her hara between your two hands by placing the palm of one over her belly and the other over her lower back. Hold until you feel a connection between your two hands. Then release.

10 Pressing the hips and down the legs

Kneel facing your partner and apply pressure to the muscles of the hips and down the exposed sides of both legs, including the feet. Keep one hand as a 'support' and use the other active hand to give pressure.

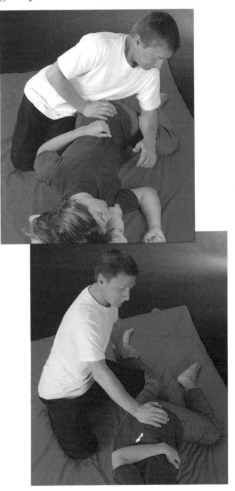

Sitting Shiatsu

Sitting Shiatsu is an especially good position for working on the upper part of the body. It can be included as part of an overall treatment or it can be given as a 'mini' boost to relax a person, for example in the middle of a busy day.

Position

Always sit your partner in a way that is most comfortable for her.

1 Sitting on the floor

Seisa

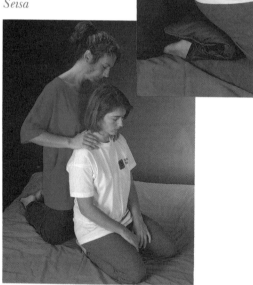

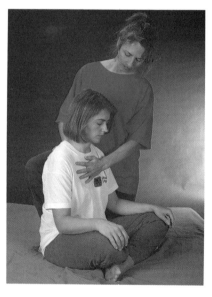

Crossed legged

Legs straight

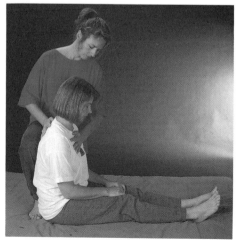

Seisa is a Japanese way of sitting between the heels with the lower legs folded under the thighs and the big toes crossed. The position is very beneficial as it stimulates the channels of the legs, thus strengthening the organs of the body. It also keeps the spine straight and head balanced which allows ease of breathing and free energy flow up the spine. Difficulty in sitting in seisa can indicate too much fluid in the legs and a weakening condition.

In any floor sitting positions:

- Sit your partner on the edge of a small cushion to increase her comfort.

- Support your partner's back whenever possible, by letting her lean against your body . . .

- or by putting one leg up, and bracing her back.

2 Sitting on a chair

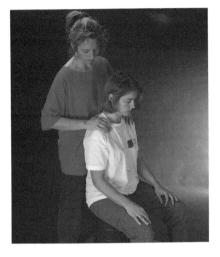

When it is more convenient or if your partner cannot easily sit on the floor let her sit on an upright chair or stool. The height must enable you to work comfortably. Again support her back when necessary.

Shiatsu technique

Take a few moments to rest your hands on your partner's shoulders and centre yourself before you begin working.

1 Scalp massage

Cup your partner's forehead in your hand and bend her head

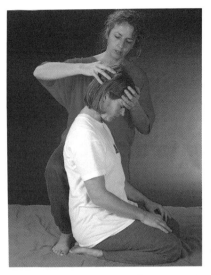

forward. Encourage her to relax and let you fully support the weight of her head in your hand. With the fingers and thumb of your free hand massage firmly and slowly all over the scalp. Move the skin over the bone and include the areas behind the ears and along the hair line. Work generously. Then support her head as you gently bring it up.

2 Head turn

Keep your partner's shoulders straight and turn her head by taking your hand around the front

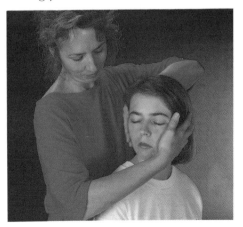

of her face to the opposite cheek and gently pulling it. Support her other cheek with your other hand to keep her head vertical. Hold the maximum stretch and slowly release. Change the position of your hands and repeat turning her head to the other side.

3 Neck stretch and roll

Stand behind your partner and support her back if necessary. Rest your elbows on her shoulders and place your hands over each other on the back of her head. Gently press it forward to the point of resistance whilst your elbows secure the shoulders and hold them back. Hold and apply comfortable pressure to stretch the back of the neck and upper body. Encourage your partner to breathe more deeply and relax into the stretch.

Then cup her forehead in your hand and slowly raise it. Securely support the back of her neck with your other hand and tilt her head back.

Now, gently and slowly, roll her head from side to side between the support of your stretched thumb and forefingers.

5 Shoulder squeeze

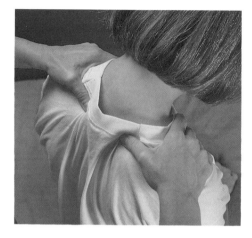

Squeeze and roll the muscles of the shoulders between your thumb and fingers. Feel for knots and tight muscles. Focus gentle yet penetrating pressure on tender areas.

Be careful not to merely pinch the skin, as this will hurt.

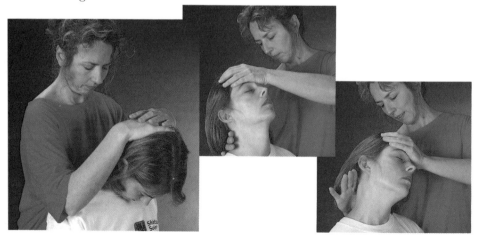

6 Rubbing and pounding the shoulder muscles and back

Stand or kneel at your partner's side and place one of your hands on her upper chest. Use the heel of your other hand to rub firmly, then rotate and vibrate the muscles of her upper back between the shoulder blades, along her back and along the top of her shoulders. Also work down the muscles either side of her spine to the sacrum. You can also use your finger and thumb tips or the whole of your palm. Change your position and work on the other side.

it. Your leg should comfortably support her upper arm horizontally. If necessary stretch out your foot to lower your leg if it holds the arm uncomfortably high.

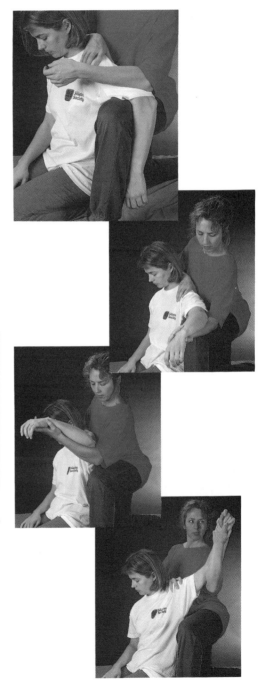

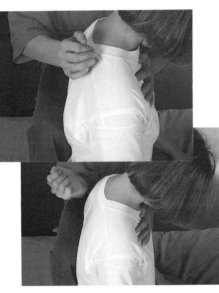

For a more vigorous stimulation stand or kneel behind your partner and pound rhythmically with loose fists, striking the muscles along the top of her shoulders and upper back.

7 Pressing and rotating the arms

Kneel behind your partner as she sits on the floor. Bend your knee up at her side and lay her arm over

Rest your support hand on her shoulder and use your forearm and then your hand to press slowly down the outside of her arm.

Now, while firmly supporting her shoulder joint, hold her wrist and rotate her arm. Keep it straight as you move it forward up and back describing a full circle. Move the position of your body to echo the rotation.

Circulate the arm 2 or 3 times. At times hold the upward and backward stretches for a few moments to open up the shoulder joint and armpit.

Release her arm and repeat the sequence on the other side.

If your partner is sitting on a chair, stand behind her, resting your foot on the side of a chair, stool or box and support her arm over your thigh.

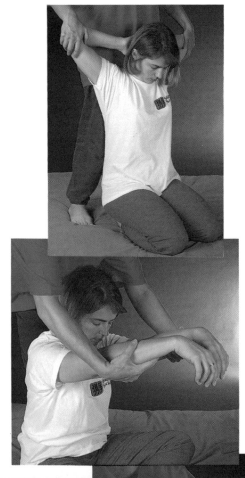

8 Arm stretches

Stand behind your partner. Ask her to clasp her hands behind her head and inhale. As she breathes out pull her elbows back, opening

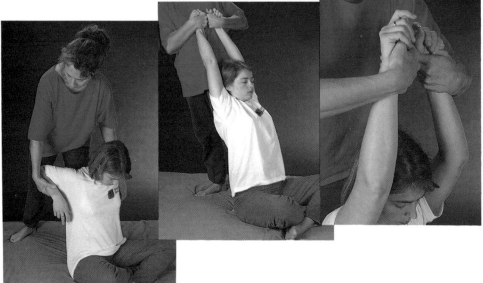

and stretching the front of her chest. Remind her to relax her neck and to let her head drop forward. Support her back if necessary.

Hold the stretch and release.

This sequence can only be given when your partner is sitting on the floor preferably cross-legged. Position the outside of your foot at the base of your partner's spine. Then stretch her arms out in front of her and up over her head. As you do this, slide your hands along her arms and clasp her wrists, or hands, firmly. Lean back and stretch her along the side of your body. Encourage her to relax fully and then release the stretch.

Now hold your partner's forearms and bend her elbows, bringing them back and up behind her. This stretches the shoulder joints in the opposite direction. Hold at maximum stretch and release.

9 Stretching the back

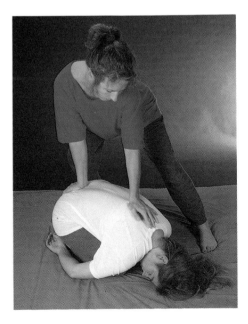

With your partner in seisa position, knees slightly open, ask her to fold her body forward between her thighs. Lay her arms by her side and turn her head to one side. If she is stiff you can place a cushion between her buttocks and heels for added comfort.

Your partner can also sit cross legged or on a chair and lean forward, supporting her elbows on her knees as you work on her back.

Stand beside your partner and rest the heel of your hand on the base of her spine, with your fingers curling over her buttocks. Place your other hand between her shoulder blades with the fingers pointing towards her head. Now stretch her spine by leaning your weight over your partner as you push your hands apart. Be sensitive to her flexibility as you press down. Hold the stretch and release.

Keep your hand resting on her sacrum and place the first 2 fingers of your other hand on either side of her spine. Vigorously rub up and down its length. Change your hand position and support the top of her back with one hand. Rub the muscles on either side of her spine with the fingers of your other hand.

In seisa position the back is fully exposed and can be rubbed, pressed, stretched and kneaded in many ways. Only work in this position for as long as your partner is comfortable and then slowly help her back to an upright position.

10 Shoulder stretch

With your partner sitting in seisa, knees slightly open, help her to stretch her arms over your thighs

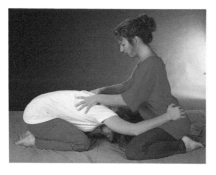

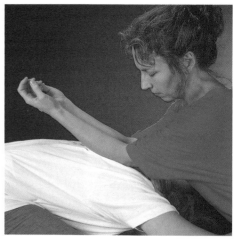

as you sit at her head. Let her relax into the stretch and then gently lean your weight into her upper back. Work from her shoulders down to her mid-back either side of the spine, using your forearm, palms and/or thumbs. Also press the muscles along the top of her shoulders.

Work with care. Gradually increase your pressure, keeping within the range of your partner's comfort and flexibility. Then help her out of the stretch, slowly.

Shiatsu given with the feet

Shiatsu given with the feet can be a deep and fulfilling experience. Your feet can become almost as sensitive as your hands and be used with great dexterity. To achieve this control and balance are essential as the legs and feet are powerful tools. Care is needed to use them with grace for they can impart a delicate touch as well as forceful pressure. Standing upright as you work allows you to press with and use your whole body weight. Strong and effective treatments can be given in this way without becoming tired.

It takes practice to give good 'barefoot' treatments: you need to be fully centred in your hara to awaken awareness in your legs and for your feet to become like 'eyes'. The use of feet in Shiatsu is an extensive study and includes advanced techniques of standing and walking on your partner (see Suggested Reading).

In this section some simple approaches only are suggested which can easily be incorporated into your treatment.

Position

Most commonly your partner will lie prone exposing the strong muscles of the back of the body that are most suitable to be worked on by the feet.

When your partner lies supine treat only the more muscular parts of her body, for example, her thighs and upper arms.

Shiatsu technique

1 Rocking

Place your foot on your partner's lower back and rock her pelvis. Allow her natural 'rock back' movement to dictate the speed and rhythm.

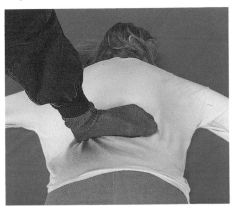

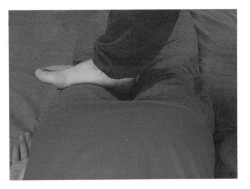

You can also roll the muscle of the thigh and upper arm when your partner lies supine.

3 Giving pressure

Balance yourself securely on your standing leg and use the ball or heel of your foot to press slowly over the muscular areas of your partner's back, arms and legs. For more dispersed weight use the flat of your foot. For increased precision press with the point of your toes.

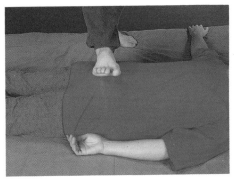

When lying supine your partner can be rocked by nudging her from the side with the ball, middle or heel of your foot.

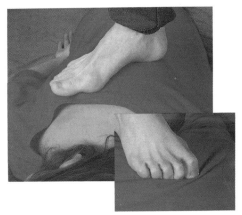

2 Rolling the muscles

Use light pressure and roll the strong muscles of the leg, upper arm and back with the sole of your foot. Balance yourself firmly on your standing leg with knee slightly bent and carefully control your use of pressure.

4 Treading on the feet

Stand between your partner's feet facing away from her. With your heels walk on the soles of her feet. Shift your weight from one foot to the other. Avoid treading on her toes as this will hurt.

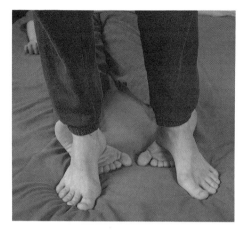

WARNING: Only tread on your partner's feet if they lie flat with no gap between ankle and floor.

5 Stimulating and relaxing the spine

Face your partner standing between her legs. Place your foot over the base of her spine (coccyx).

Use your heel to push it quickly, letting its movement create a rhythm. You should see her whole spine and head move.

Stand beside your partner's shoulder and place the ball of your foot on her sacrum. Press down and towards her feet. Hold and release.

6 Loosening the shoulders

Sit with your legs at each side of your partner's head and place your feet on her shoulders. Then rhythmically press the muscles of each shoulder alternately. Use the ball of your foot, the arch or heel to give pressure moving the position of your feet from her neck out towards the shoulder joints.

This treatment can also be given when your partner is lying on her back.

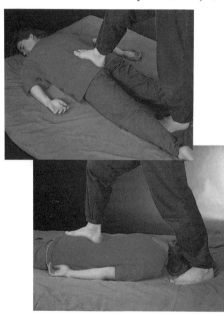

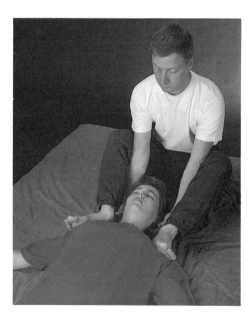

Finishing off and after the treatment

The way you conclude a treatment and leave your partner is important as this remains foremost in her mind. A good Shiatsu can be marred by a rough or inconclusive ending. In the same way that you approach and start a treatment gently, you should also leave your partner softly and in peace.

Allow at least 5 to 10 minutes for your partner to relax after the massage. This gives her body a chance to assimilate and feel the benefits of your touch. It is important for your partner to gather herself slowly, without rushing. Be clear with your partner especially if she is new to Shiatsu. Speak quietly and tell her in your own way that the treatment has ended and that she can lie and relax for a few minutes before getting up.

Ways to finish off

Suggested here are connecting movements, and areas to hold at the end of a treatment. They can be used individually, or combined in a way that you feel will suit the needs of your partner and leave her with a sense of wholeness.

1 Brushing

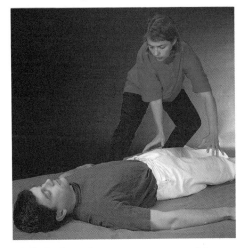

Lightly brush your partner with a feather touch on the surface of his skin or just above, keeping your wrists loose and hands relaxed. Focus on your hands as you do this and be centred.

Your partner can lie prone or supine, be sitting or standing.

'Brushing up' the body has a stimulating effect and should be done from the hips and up and right off the top of the head. 'Brushing down' the body, working from above the head and down and off the feet, is more soothing.

2 Resting hand

Sit close to your partner and place one hand on the part of her body which feels weak or in need. This often will be the heart centre (front chest, or the upper back) or the hara (belly or small of the back). Let your other hand rest on your knee, palm upper most. Relax your shoulders and deepen your breathing and have your awareness on your hands. After a time, slowly take your hand away.

3 Connecting points

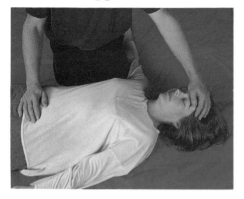

Use both your hands lightly to hold and connect points and areas of the body. Be relaxed and fully focused in both hands and centred in yourself as you do this. The aim is to encourage balance in your partner, so you want to connect opposite, or diagonally opposite, parts of her body. For example:

- Use one hand on the upper body (above the waist) and one hand on the lower body.

- Rest one hand on the right side and your other hand on the left side of the spine.

- Use one hand on the back and your other hand on the front of her body.

- Rest your hands on both her feet.

Also resting your hands on any two of the centre line chakras (see page 138) can feel good and be beneficial.

Finally, cover your partner with a blanket unless it is extremely warm, before leaving her to relax. She may feel chilly because being inactive in a deeply relaxed state causes the body temperature to drop.

Re-centering yourself

Cleansing yourself of your partner's energy and influence after a treatment is important. It takes only a few moments and can be done as your partner relaxes.

1 Washing your hands

Wash your hands and arms up to the elbows in water and shake off. If you don't have access to water simply perform the motions of washing, brushing and shaking imaginary water off your arms and hands.

2 Clearing your Aura

Stand squarely with your knees slightly bent.

1 Use the fingers of both your hands together and lightly trace along the centre line of your body beginning between your eyebrows. Slowly move up and over your head to the back of your neck.

2 Now take one hand, reach around your face and using your palm, smooth down the side and back of the neck, shoulders, arm, hand and off the finger tips. Repeat this with your other hand, smoothing down the other side.

3 Now take your finger tips as high up your back as you can reach and brush down the spine to the base. Use your palms to fan out over the buttocks and down the back of each leg and off the feet.

4 Then smooth down the front of the body with your finger tips meeting at the centre line. Begin on your face or throat, using the flat of your hand over your chest,

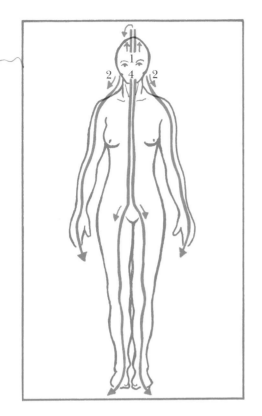 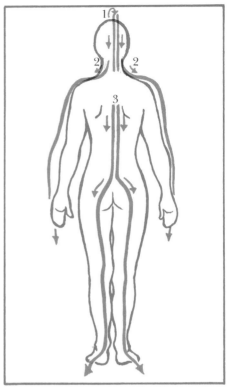

abdomen, groin and down the front and inside of each leg and off the feet.

Make your movements slowly with full awareness and attention. Work to the very end of your extremities and off. After smoothing each part of your body flick your hands into a corner as though you are shaking off excess energy. This sequence takes no more than one minute.

And finally

Share your experience of the treatment with your partner and discuss any observations that you made. Suggest exercises and changes in diet or lifestyle that she can make to improve and strengthen her condition. Also encourage her to give you her feelings and comments on the treatment.

3

THE BASIC SEQUENCE

Forming a treatment

Your Shiatsu treatment can take any form. The various techniques can be used and put together in different ways to suit the individual needs of your partner.

The important thing is to become familiar in using the techniques and become confident in moving and handling a partner's body. Smooth transition from one part of the body to another is essential. This comes with practice and means that you must be flexible and agile enough to move comfortably around your partner. Don't move your partner unnecessarily and let your Shiatsu become like a dance as each technique flows into the next.

If you sense that your partner is shy or lacks confidence about receiving Shiatsu, begin your treatment on her back. She will feel less vulnerable when she lies prone and will be able to relax more easily. As a beginner it can also be easier to begin your treatment on the back.

However, as your confidence and skill develop you can begin your Shiatsu treatment on the front of the body and make an initial hara diagnosis. Use this as a treatment guide. At the end of a treatment again diagnose the hara to see what changes have taken place and the effectiveness of your Shiatsu.

Things to remember

- Always centre yourself before you begin.

- Make a general plan of your treatment and run it through your mind. Keep it simple.

- There is no rush. Anxiety makes us move faster and want to put more into a treatment. You can work more slowly and hold areas for longer. This will give a more penetrating treatment.

- If you forget, feel confused or unsure of what to do next, simply pause. Rest your hands on your partner as you centre yourself and gather your thoughts. Continue when you're ready.

- At any time be prepared to adjust your treatment in response to new information that you gather as you work. Be aware of the diagnostic points and areas (see pages 128–130). Also notice the condition of the channels, tsubos and kyo jitsu balance.

Suggested sequence

This sequence is basic. Techniques can be added to it. For example if your partner has lower back trouble extra stretches can be added that may relieve and strengthen the area.

Your audio cassette also goes through this sequence with you.

Lie your partner prone

1   *Sit beside her, centre yourself and make contact.* (page 29)

2   *Gently begin to rock her hips.* (page 34)

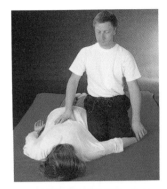

Come up onto your knees facing your partner

3   *'Baby Walk' over her back.* (page 35)

4   *Give diagonal stretches.* (pages 36–37)

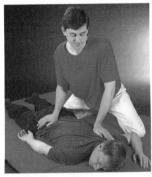

Keep one hand on her sacrum as you move to kneel above her head

5   *Place both hands on her sacrum and stretch.* (page 37)

6   *Use the heel of your hands and your thumbs to press along her shoulder muscles and down her upper back.* (page 36)

7   *Slide both palms down her back to her sacrum, pressing the heels into the muscles.*

8   *Stretch her sacrum again.* (page 37)

9   *Lightly draw your hands up her back and neck and off her head.*

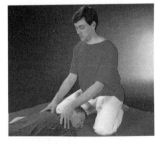

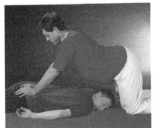

Keep one hand resting on your partner's upper back as you move and kneel by her other side

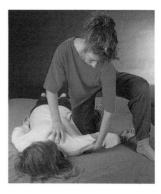

10 *Loosen her shoulder and her arm next to you.* (page 52)

11 *Work around her shoulder blade.* (page 58)

Release her arm and stand astride your partner facing her head

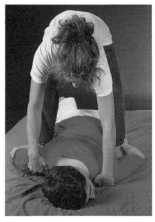

12 *Lift and shake both shoulders.* (page 57)

Step over to the other side of your partner's body and kneel

13 *Loosen your partner's shoulder and down her arm.* (page 52)

14 *Work around her shoulder blade.* (page 58)

Release her arm

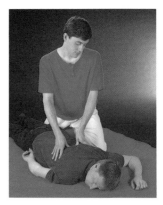

15 *Use the sides of your hands to 'saw' up and down the muscles of her back.* (page 34)

16 *Apply thumb pressure down her back.* (page 35)

17 *Press her sacrum.* (pages 39–40)

18 *Squeeze her hips.* (page 40)

19 *Palm down the back of her straight leg.* (page 46)

20 *Bend her leg pressing the heel to her buttocks.* (pages 46–47)

21 *Kidney Palm heal.* (page 50)

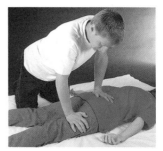

Stand and pick up her other leg

22 Achilles tendon stretch.

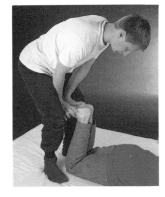

Release her first leg. Position yourself on the opposite side of your partner

23 Bend her other leg and press the heel to her buttocks. (pages 46–47)

24 Kidney Palm heal on this side. (page 50)

25 Straighten her leg and palm down the back of it. (page 46)

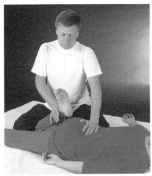

Move to your partner's feet

26 Walk on the soles of her feet. (pages 75–76)

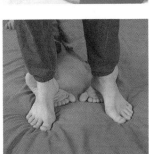

Help your partner turn over (page 33)

Lie your partner supine (page 33)

1 Hold her hara. (pages 43–44)

2 Create a 'wave' movement on her hara. (page 44)

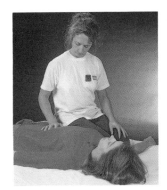

3 Palm and thumb down the front of her leg.
(pages 47–48)

4 Rotate and stretch the leg. (page 41)

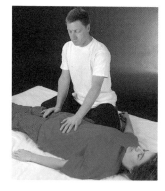

5 Twist your partner. (page 38) Release slowly and
straighten her leg.

6 Bend her leg out to the side and give pressure down
the inside. (pages 48–49)

Straighten your leg as you move to her feet

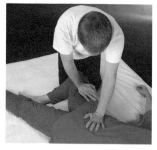

Then kneel beside her foot

7 Thoroughly press and rotate her foot.
(page 51)

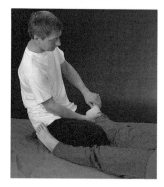

Stand up and take hold of both feet

8 Stretch both legs. (page 49)

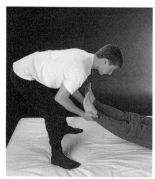

Release the first leg and move to the other side
of your partner

Kneel beside her foot

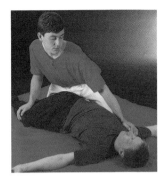

9   *Thoroughly press and rotate her foot.* (page 51)

10 *Rotate and stretch her leg.* (page 41)

11 *Twist your partner.* (page 38)

12 *Bend her leg out to the side and give pressure down the inside.* (pages 48–49)

Stand astride your partner at hip level facing her head

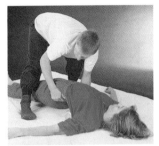

13 *Roll her hips.* (page 42)

Then move to kneel at her side

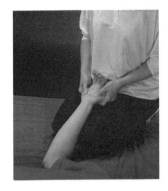

14 *Press on the shoulder next to you and palm down her arm.* (page 53)

15 *Press her hand.* (page 53)

Step to position yourself behind her head

16 *Stretch her arm over her head.* (page 54)

Move and pick up her other arm

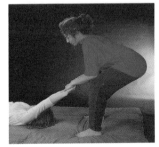

17 *Stretch both arms.* (page 54)

Release her first arm

18 *Stretch her other arm over her head.* (page 54)

Step and re-position yourself by her other side

19 *Press down on her shoulder and palm down her arm.* (page 53)

20 *Press her hand.* (page 53)

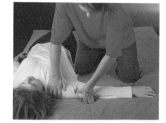

Rest your fingers on her chest and move to kneel behind your partner's head

21 *Press down on her chest.* (page 56)

22 *Check the back of her neck.* (page 60)

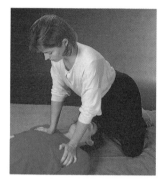

23 *Press into her neck and around the base of her skull. Massage her scalp.* (page 62)

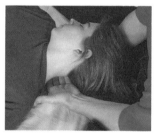

Gently centre your partner's head

24 *Run your fingers through her hair.* (page 62)

25 *Relax her face.* (page 62)

26 *Relax the back of her neck again.* (page 60)

27 *Finish off by connecting and holding points.* (page 78)

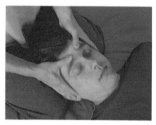

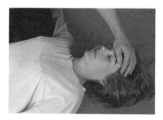

Slowly release and draw your hands off your partner.

4
PRACTICAL GUIDELINES

> **❝** *If one is sick of sickness then one is not sick.* **❞**
> Lau Tzu

Reaction situations

Shiatsu gives most people a feeling of lightness, relaxation, renewed energy and well-being. Over a period of regular treatments medical symptoms can often be relieved. However, at times uncomfortable responses can occur during and after a treatment. This is rare, but in giving Shiatsu you need to be aware of the possibility of reactions.

Understanding the reactions

Your Shiatsu treatment will stimulate the movement of energy in a person and begin to activate stagnant or blocked Ki. As this happens the body will begin to remove accumulated toxins from the system and it is this movement that creates symptoms such as tiredness, headaches, nausea, joint pains, aching muscles, rashes and emotional sensitivity. These temporary discomforts, although very unpleasant, need not be cause for concern. In fact such reactions indicate that the body is cleansing itself and healing is taking place.

Reaction symptoms only happen when the body is eliminating toxins and as such they indicate a positive change in a person's condition. They will be most noticeable in people new to Shiatsu, especially if they have not had other forms of body work or have not taken much care of themselves. The natural response of the body is to cleanse itself. These reactions and symptoms will lessen with subsequent Shiatsu treatments as the body becomes more balanced and healthy.

Reactions will usually appear some hours after a treatment and last for about one day.

The symptoms are generally physically orientated although emotional feelings can also surface. They may be mild or more acute.

What to do

- In a reassuring way tell newcomers to Shiatsu of the possibility of experiencing these reactions and why.

- Suggest that they allow the reaction to run its course without interference as it is part of the healing process.

- Be available for them to telephone you in case they need reassurance or want to talk.

When Shiatsu should not be given

There are times when Shiatsu is not appropriate and for certain conditions it can be harmful:

- in conditions of contagious illness or disease;

- if there is the possibility of blood clots, threat of internal bleeding or twisted intestine;

- if there is cancer, as there is a theoretical risk that heavy, dispersing-style Shiatsu may stimulate circulation of cancer cells;

- with high fever;

- with an infectious skin condition present or on acne, rashes and open cuts;

- over swellings, bruises and sprains;

- over local inflammation and infection;

- over areas of excessive tenderness and pain;

- on broken bones;

- on varicose veins;

- on the ankles or lower legs during pregnancy as pressure on these areas can induce miscarriage;

- directly on top of the shoulders (tsubo GB21) during pregnancy as pressure on this area can induce miscarriage (see page 94).

A final word

A degree of common sense and a realistic acceptance of your own limitations is needed when you give Shiatsu.

Remember that you are not an expert yet. Although Shiatsu can treat more serious conditions this should only be attempted by an experienced Shiatsu specialist in consultation with a doctor. Shiatsu is primarily preventative health care and when you use it in this way you will have success and gain valuable experience.

Touch is healing and comforting. When Shiatsu cannot be directly used on an area, for example when there is acute pain, an open wound, broken bones and so on, you can give palm healing (see page 24). Unaffected parts of the body can also be held or touched softly and gently stroked to reassure and ease tension.

5

SPECIAL CIRCUMSTANCES

> *" A tree that is unbending is easily broken. "*
> Lau Tzu

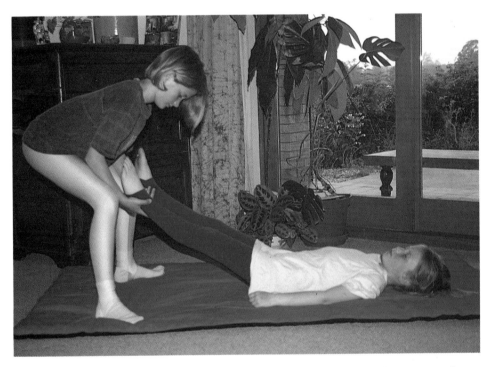

Shiatsu is not just for the specialist or the health fanatic. It is open and available for all to use. It is simply touch and as such it is a wonderful and enjoyable form of communication, of giving and receiving.

In Japan Shiatsu is integrated into daily life and commonly practised in the family. Both the elderly and the very young receive Shiatsu and it is an excellent way of helping pregnant women enjoy their condition. Those who are physically active such as dancers, sports people, manual labourers, will all appreciate the value of Shiatsu. In different ways physically inactive people, such as desk workers and those who are disabled or bed-ridden, also benefit tremendously from Shiatsu stimulation.

The approach and techniques of Shiatsu are varied and flexible. With common sense and an empathy for your partner Shiatsu can easily be adapted to suit differing needs and specific circumstances. Some guidelines are given here.

Shiatsu for the young

In many cultures massaging babies and young children is seen as an essential part of their upbringing.

Shiatsu can be given to the very young and it has many benefits:

- it is fun and pleasurable;

- it encourages bonding and closeness between adult/parent and child;

- it promotes health, emotional well-being and physical and mental development;

- it gives opportunities for the adult/parent to notice early any physical abnormalities and misalignments, which can then be corrected or professional help sought.

Things to remember

- **Make it fun.** Only do what pleases and is enjoyable. Stop at any sign of discomfort or discontent in your baby or child.

- **Use less pressure.** Be very aware of the size, delicacy and sensitivity of the little person you are touching.

- **Be relaxed and unhurried.** This is very important.

- **Remember: your baby or child's concentration span is short.** Plan short frequent sessions. A complete Shiatsu can be divided into sections and given at different times during the day.

- **Be flexible.** Your baby or child will wriggle and want to move so adapt your treatment and follow their lead.

- **Make the room very warm and comfortable**

Babies

Pleasurable touch and tactile stimulation is vital for the healthy development of babies. Gentle manipulation and movement of their joints and limbs also stimulates balanced growth and brain development.

How to start

Massage your baby naked and have the room very warm. Direct skin contact is stimulating, reassuring and pleasurable. Touch the different parts of your baby as you hold him or lie him on your knees, on a warm surface or comfortably on the floor. Make sure the baby is well supported and can't fall. Be prepared to change positions frequently as he wriggles and wants to move.

Tactile stimulation

Vary your approach and at times massage with powder or a little warm oil. (Choose a vegetable oil such as almond.)

Also brush your baby's skin with a baby brush, soft cloth or the back of a warm spoon for extra stimulation.

Technique

Begin gently touching and stroking your baby from birth. Don't have set ideas or a programme, simply enjoy the sensations and getting to know each other.

As you both become used to a massaging touch and as your baby grows older, begin to introduce aspects of Shiatsu in a relaxed way.

- **Stroke along the channels.**

- **Stimulate all the channels** each day.

- **Massage** the back, feet, hands, ears and hara.

- **Stretch** and move the limbs and encourage flexibility of the joints and spine.

Young children

As your baby becomes a toddler and grows into a child, your Shiatsu can become more specific.

Technique

Begin tracing the channels, using light thumb pressure.

Work with the general principles of Shiatsu and make the massage as interesting and enjoyable as you can. Be inventive.

As your child becomes older and his attention span increases, you can reduce the number of sessions and make them longer. Also include exercise along with the massage. However, still keep some sessions for massage alone with the emphasis on relaxation for those times when your child is tired or needs to calm down. This will help him to understand about relaxation and give him a means to do it on his own.

Exercise

During the Shiatsu, stretch and rotate the limbs, giving a gentle twist to the spine and begin simple 'acrobatics-type' exercises. Children love being handled, turned upside down, walking on their hands and so on, as long as they are very securely held and feel safe. The idea is not to do 'dare devil' stunts, but simply to stretch joints and channels, encourage circulation and develop flexibility.

Your child will grow in confidence as he gets to know his body and experiences his capabilities.

Teach your child Shiatsu

As soon as your child has dexterity and shows an interest, encourage him to touch and massage. Children are naturally curious, co-operative and love to give. Let them be important and make you feel good.

Show them how to massage your feet, stroke your face, squeeze your shoulder and walk on your back – something that can be great fun and feel good.

Difficult children

Some children are difficult, very unco-operative and extremely hard to handle and communicate with, to the extent of being disturbed and in need of special help.

Even so, give them massage, encourage them to exercise and make them the centre of your attention. They may oppose and reject you, but lovingly persist, without criticism, anger or force. It can be fun after all and what child will always refuse a call to play?

Also encourage them to massage, to give to others, to feel involved and be part of what is happening. Be infinitely patient and, who knows, you may be pleasantly surprised at how well your child eventually responds.

Shiatsu for the elderly

In later life, the amount of caring touch that we receive tends to lessen and unfortunately for many people, it can become virtually non-existent.

Moreover, this happens at a time when stiffness, aches and pains could be relieved with a tender touch; the ageing body is appreciative of the nourishment of contact.

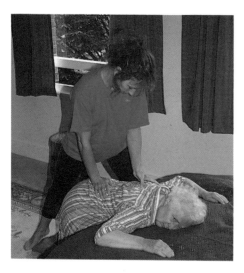

Approach

Shiatsu can be lightly given, and is easily adjusted to suit a frail form, or inflexible joints. An appreciation of your partner's condition and fragility is essential as you give your treatment. Many older people are robust and in good health. Even so, a gentle approach is necessary, as bones and ligaments are likely to be more brittle, flexibility limited and the processes of the body slowed down.

Position

Treat your partner in whichever position is most comfortable for her. Be inventive if she is stiff and has restricted movement.

This may be seated in a chair as many people will not want, or will not be able, to get down on the floor.

If available, your partner can lie on a very firm bed, or on a massage table. This will restrict some of your Shiatsu technique, but the convenience of it makes it worthwhile.

Whatever position your partner is in, ensure her comfort by using cushions to ease discomfort or stiffness. Make sure that you can freely and comfortably move around her.

Points to remember

- **Use less pressure** and less forceful manipulations. Palm healing can be effective and appropriate (see page 24).

- **Don't massage inflamed (arthritic) joints.** When there is no inflammation, massage can be beneficial.

- **Concentrate on the extremities.** Circulation may be poor and hand, foot and lower leg treatment can be especially helpful.

- **Rotate joints and stretch limbs**, keeping well within your partner's mobility and pain threshold range.

- **Keep your partner comfortable** and make sure she moves frequently, to avoid the onset of stiffness.

- **Keep the room extra warm** and a blanket handy to cover your partner should she become cold.

- **Remain very aware** and sensitive to your partner's needs and her reaction to your touch.

Shiatsu in pregnancy

In recent years, natural childbirth has grown in popularity and more women are eager to give birth without drugs or forceps.

In Japan Shiatsu traditionally has been used to help women in pregnancy, to assist during labour and the birth and afterwards to promote the necessary body contractions. It is also recommended for those women wishing to become pregnant; teamed with good nutrition and regular exercise, Shiatsu can improve the health and emotional well-being of the mother-to-be. In this way the optimum conditions are encouraged for conception and the growth of the baby.

Benefits

Shiatsu strengthens the internal organs and systems of the body and improves flexibility of muscles, ligaments and joints in preparation for birth.

- It can help relieve common discomforts, such as backache, tiredness, nausea, constipation, headaches, stress and tension (see pages 97–101).

- It offers a way for the mother-to-be to become more intimately acquainted with her body, how it works and how it feels.

- It will encourage contact with her growing baby and begin the bonding process in the womb.

- As the father of the child gives her Shiatsu, he will feel included and involved in the wonderful growing process of his baby.

- The growing baby will also be stimulated by the Shiatsu treatments.

Approach

Shiatsu, given with sensitivity and care, can be very supportive and helpful in easing the aches and pains of pregnancy. Work gently with a certain delicacy and respect for the condition of your partner. Ask her to tell you what feels good, what she wants and when your pressure is too strong or inappropriate.

Technique

There are two major aspects to note in giving Shiatsu during pregnancy:

1 Specific tsubos are traditionally avoided

These are said to promote miscarriage and pressure should not be given to them (see illustration).

As a general rule, avoid giving pressure anywhere on the ankles or lower leg. The area around the ankles corresponds to the sexual organs and pressure can stimulate activity there.

Also, avoid giving Shiatsu to the shoulder muscles (notably GB21),

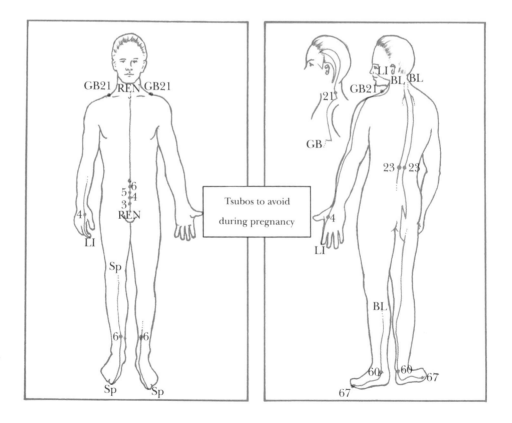

Tsubos to avoid during pregnancy

or on the hand point (L14) between the thumb and index finger. Gently squeezing the shoulder muscles is acceptable.

Overall, it is better to give light dispersing-style Shiatsu rather than sustained pressure on specific tsubos during pregnancy.

2 Give side, supine, or sitting Shiatsu

Lying prone quickly becomes unsuitable for pregnant women as they begin to swell. Side Shiatsu is particularly comfortable and allows access to all parts of your partner's body.

Things to remember

- **Ensure your partner's comfort.** Use cushions to ease strain and prop her body.

- **Listen to your partner** and follow her lead.

- **Work with care and gentleness.** Avoid rough or vigorous techniques and prolonged pressure on tsubos.

- **Only use palm healing** on hara, lower legs and ankles.

Ways to prepare for the birth

Babies come slowly and the 9 month gestation period is the time for both mother and father to prepare for the birth and for welcoming a new soul into this world.

- **Practise Shiatsu techniques with your partner** and become familiar and well acquainted with her body, and its individuality.

- **Through Shiatsu exercise, quiet contemplation and meditation**, the mother-to-be can come to know herself more fully, and have confidence in her ability to give birth.

- **Understand the physical changes taking place** as the baby grows and prepares to be born. Know about what to expect during labour and birth. This will help reduce fears and anxieties.

- **Join one of the very good pre-natal classes.**

Shiatsu and the birth

Shiatsu can be used effectively during the birth process to ease pain and promote the delivery. Remember to talk to your doctor and midwife about the kind of birth you both want. You need to have their understanding and co-operation if you want to use Shiatsu.

Birth is a unique experience and even with full preparation and participation it may not happen in the way that you both imagine. If Shiatsu does not give you the results you hoped for during the birth, remember that your love, care and presence as you support and help your partner and baby in the birth process will be invaluable to them.

Shiatsu for common ailments

An overall view of the body and the interrelationship of its organs, systems and function is important.

In understanding sickness there is a tendency to look no further than the symptoms and, in a superficial and erroneous way, think these to be the cause of the problem.

For example, a woman experiencing weak and tender ankles may well think that the ankle joints are to blame, and try to treat them accordingly. Meanwhile the deeper relationship of the ankles to the whole body, and their specific connection to the reproductive organs is overlooked and consequently the possibility that a problem in the uterus or ovaries is the primary cause of the weak ankles.

Treating the symptoms can bring relief, but it will not affect the underlying cause of a condition. However, sometimes symptomatic relief is very welcome and extremely helpful as a short term solution.

Basic principles of treatment

- Firstly, relax your partner. Stress is a major cause of many problems and the discomfort or pain of the symptoms in themselves will create tension in her body. If time permits, a full Shiatsu treatment is always a good idea.

- Press tsubos related to the problem area.

- Give Shiatsu to the channel(s) flowing through the problem area.

- Give Shiatsu to the channel directly affected by a condition.

- Give Shiatsu to the opposite side of the body to the problem area:
  Side to side, for example, when the left shoulder is extremely painful, work on the right shoulder first.
  Top to bottom, for example, headaches can sometimes be relieved by working on the feet.

Lower back pain can be eased by thoroughly relaxing the muscles and vertebrae of the neck.
Back to front, for example, deep Shiatsu given to the hara can lessen lower backache.

- Initially work indirectly in the ways suggested above before directly approaching the affected area. Give Shiatsu only if the area is not inflamed, an open wound or too painful to touch (see counter indications page 88).

- When in doubt, give palm healing.

Specific conditions

There are many good books on how to treat common problems/ ailments (see Suggested Reading list, page 143). The list of disorders that can be helped is extensive, and a few examples are given here.

Headaches

Most headaches are a symptom of disorders in other parts of the body and have different causes, for example sinus congestion, digestive disorders and over indulgence, toothache, eye problems, menstrual imbalances, tension and stress.

Consequently there are many types of headaches which affect different parts of the head. All of them produce tension or tightness in the muscles of the shoulders, neck and head.

Shiatsu is usually successful in bringing relief to headaches. However some types are persistent. If a headache constantly reoccurs despite regular Shiatsu, seek advice from your Doctor.

Basic principles of treatment

- Give Shiatsu to the upper back, shoulder, neck and head (see pages 36, 57, 59, 62).

- Also work on the extremities – hands (page 52), lower legs (avoid during pregnancy) (page 45) and especially, the feet (page 49).

- Press directly on the affected area and localised points.

Useful tsubos

Press localised points around the head, face, neck and shoulders, according to the position of the headache.

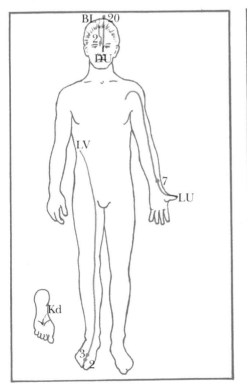

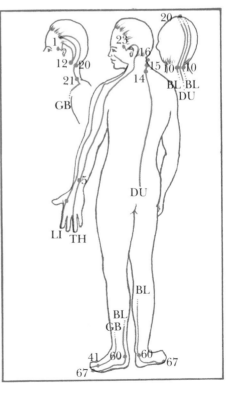

Press tsubos on the extremities such as LI4, ST36, SP6, LV2. (LI4 and SP6 are contraindicated in pregnancy.)

Migraine-type headaches

These affect specific areas of the head, with extreme pain, and have other symptoms such as nausea, impaired vision, dizziness and neck pain.

- Support your partner's head with one hand and use the other to apply strong palm pressure on the painful area for up to 10 seconds. This can be repeated as desired.

- Give firm thumb pressure, in lines approximately one inch apart, over the painful area.

Constipation and diarrhoea

These two conditions are created by the malfunctioning of the same system. This means that they respond to similar treatment, although they show very different symptoms.

The cause of constipation and diarrhoea is usually poor diet, or stress and emotional tension. Frequent Shiatsu, given over a period, can improve these conditions. When inappropriate diet is the cause, then the eating habits of a person must also be changed.

Shiatsu has very little effect when diarrhoea is caused by tainted food or bacteria.

Do not apply deep hara Shiatsu if you suspect ulcers, internal bleeding or your partner has abdominal pain.

Principles of treatment

- Work on your partner's head, neck and shoulders, down the bladder channel and feet, to release stress and ease tension.

- Concentration on her lower back and pelvis.

- Especially with constipation, massage her abdomen thoroughly until the muscles relax and the area softens.

- Treat related channels.

Lower back Shiatsu

- Use the heel of your hand to rub firmly in circular movements over her lumbar spine and sacrum. Rest your support hand on her upper back.

- Press firmly down each side of the lumbar spine. Press in the hollows of the sacrum and along both edges of the bone. (see pages 39–40)

- Work along the top of the pelvic bone and thoroughly knead her hips and buttocks. (see pages 39–40)

Useful tsubos

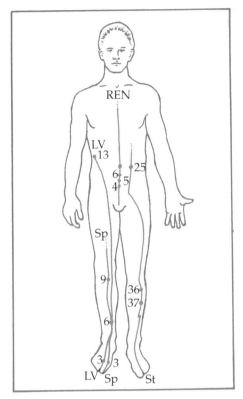

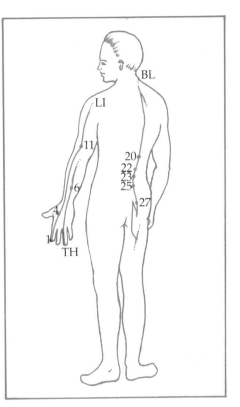

Abdomen Shiatsu

- Give deep hara Shiatsu (see pages 43–45).

- Give pressure around the abdominal area, moving up the right side of your partner and down the left (this follows the flow of the colon).

- Concentrate on tight areas, and massage until soft.

- Give leg rotations and stretches (see pages 40–42, 49).

Nausea and indigestion

Eating and drinking too much, or the wrong things, will often cause nausea and indigestion as well as stress and tension.

However, there are many other causes, including pregnancy (morning sickness), travel (motion sickness) and the malfunctioning of vital organs such as the liver, gall bladder, pancreas and heart. Inflammation of the appendix or bladder and disturbances in the digestive system can all create these symptoms.

Shiatsu can help alleviate the discomfort and unpleasant feelings; you may also need to adjust your diet.

Seek advice from your doctor if you suspect a more serious cause of your symptoms.

Basic principles of treatment

- Give Shiatsu to the head, neck, shoulders and feet to relax your partner.

- Treat related channels and give strong leg Shiatsu (stimulating Stomach, Spleen and Gall Bladder channels).

- Work slowly and sensitively on the affected area to disperse Ki. Also use palm healing.

- Work on the back stomach area.

Technique

- Place your other hand opposite it, on the back and to the left side of his spine.

- Hold, keeping yourself centered and aware. Visualise energy moving out of your hands.

- Then slowly begin to circulate your hand on the skin surface over the left side of his back up the spine and down the outside.

- Continue for some minutes.

- Bring your hand to rest again and hold before releasing.

1 Holding stomach area

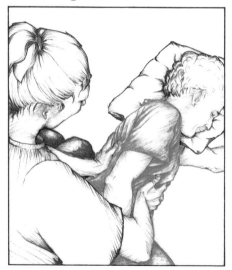

- Kneel behind your partner as he lies on his right side.

- Place your palm over the front of his stomach (cover the end of the breast bone and edge of the ribs on his left side).

2 Pressing back stomach area

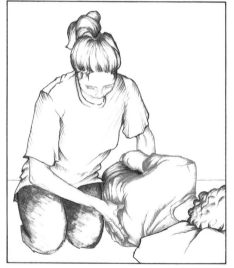

- Keep your support hand on the front of his stomach.

- Use your thumb to press deeply down the muscles on the left side of his spine from the mid-shoulder blade to just below the shoulder point.

- Work slowly and strongly and repeat 2 or 3 times.

3 Hara Shiatsu

- Concentrate on the upper hara.

- Rub the stomach area with the heel of your hand, as firmly as your partner can take.

- Press gently and deeply under the ribs beginning at the centre position and working out to both sides.

- As you work your support hand can be on the lower hara, chest, over the ribs or over the back stomach area.

4 Pressing stomach channel

- Kneel beside your partner lying supine. Place your support hand over the stomach area and use your other hand to palm down the stomach channel.

- Press and hold ST36 and use your thumb to give pressure down the lower leg.

- Then stretch her foot with your hand as you continue to hold ST36.
  Repeat 2 or 3 times. Work on the other leg in the same way.

Useful tsubos

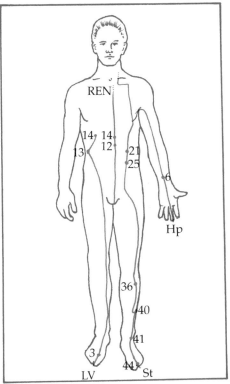

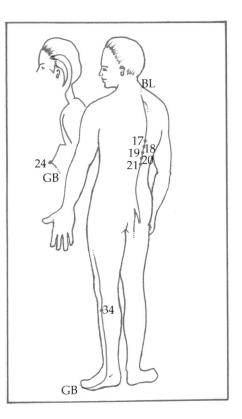

6

SELF SHIATSU

> **❝** *Let life ripen and then fall. Force is not the way at all.* **❞**
> Lau Tzu

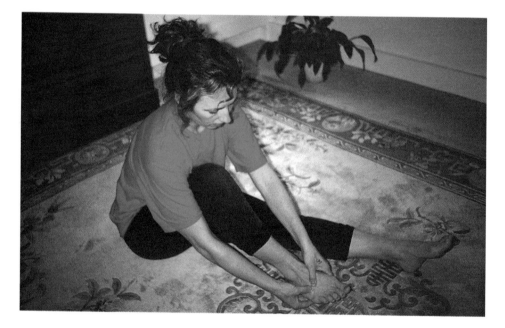

You can give Shiatsu to yourself. To do this on a regular basis is a wonderful way of maintaining health. It will also improve your knowledge and familiarity with channels and tsubos and how they function. Self Shiatsu can develop your sensitivity of touch and increase your body awareness.

The routine suggested here is basic and can be performed daily. It takes only 10 minutes. Elaborate and extend it to suit your own needs and available time by adapting any of the Shiatsu techniques to use on yourself. You are only restricted in this by your own flexibility and physical limitations.

Self Shiatsu can be done standing, sitting (on a chair, or on the floor) or lying on your back, side and to a limited extent, front.

Things to remember

- **Remain relaxed.** There will be a tendency to tense and you will need to relax consciously throughout your treatment. It is important to keep your working hand and fingers relaxed as well as the part of your body that you are treating.

- **Be comfortable.** Choose positions that are most suitable and make it easy for you to reach the part of your body you are treating.

- **Be centered** and move from your hara (see page 26).

- **Use your body weight** and lean into the pressure (see page 14).

- **Remember to breath!** Give pressure on your out breath.

- And importantly **don't rush.**

Whole body treatment

You can perform your own treatment either standing or sitting.

Head

Massage and squeeze all over your scalp (see page 62).

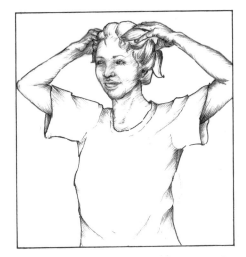

With loose fists, lightly pound over your scalp and down the back of your neck.

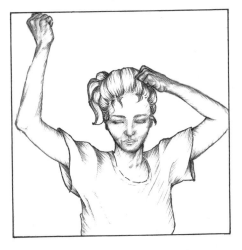

Face

Smooth the skin outwards and
upwards with your fingers (see
page 62).
   Trace the contours and press
tsubos (see page 63).

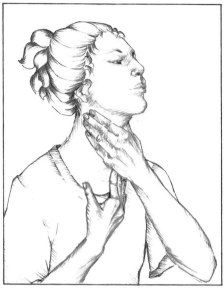

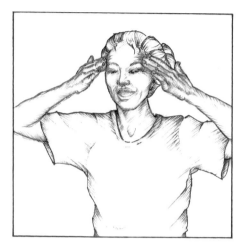

Turn your head to stretch the
side of your neck and lightly
pound up and down the
muscles . . .

Neck

Press under the rim of your skull
(see page 60).

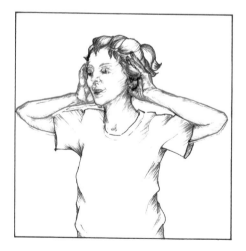

Gently stroke and squeeze the
front of your neck with the thumb
and fingers of one hand.

Shoulders

. . . and continue onto the top of
the shoulders. Reach around to the
back, and also across the front and
top of your chest. Concentrate on
tender points and muscles and
squeeze them between your thumb
and finger. Then . . .

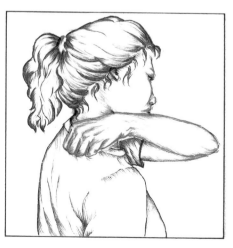

Arm

. . . continue pounding down your inside arm onto your palm.

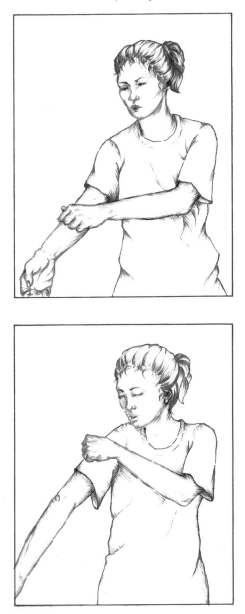

Turn your arm and pound up the outside, back to your shoulder. Repeat this 2 or 3 times.

You can also squeeze your arm, tracing the channels with your thumb and fingers.

Hand

Squeeze your hand down to the finger tips. Press the centre of your palm and the flesh between your thumb and index finger.

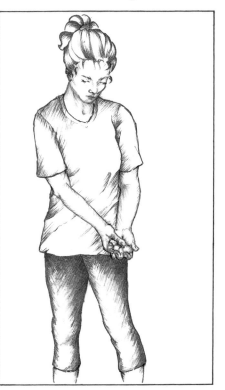

Then shake your whole arm vigorously from your shoulder. Repeat the sequence on the other side.

Stand up, if you are not already doing so . . .

Back

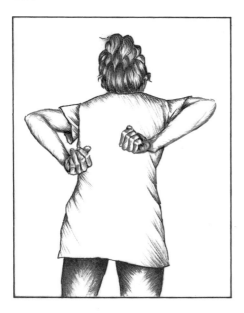

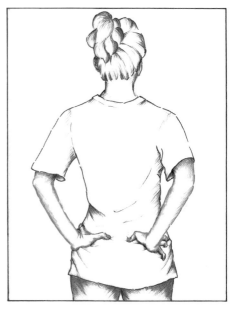

Reach both fists as high up your back as you can and pound down the muscles either side of the spine.

Press your lower back and your sacrum with your thumbs (see page 39).

Hips

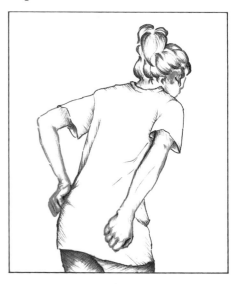

Pound over the muscles of the hips and buttocks and . . .

Legs

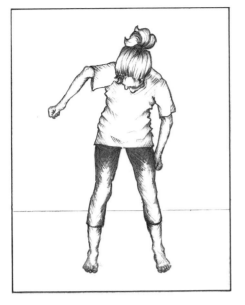

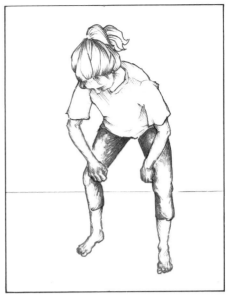

. . . continue down the outside and back of both legs.

Work up the inside. Then again down the outside. Repeat 2 or 3 times.

Now sit . . .

Hara

Bend forward slightly and sink your fingers into your hara (see page 43).

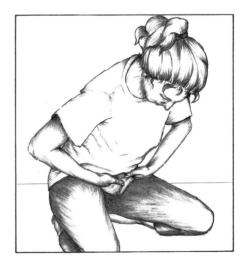

Have your legs in front of you, bend one . . .

Feet

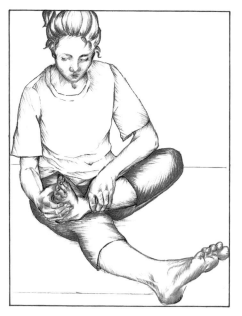

Press points on your foot and squeeze and rotate your toes (see pages 49–51).
Repeat the sequence on the other leg and foot.

. . . rotate and squeeze around your ankle.

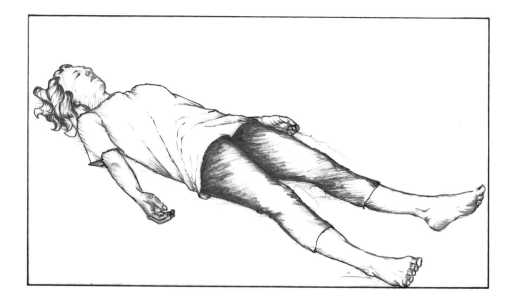

When you complete the sequence always lie on your back and relax for some minutes.

7

MAINTAINING HEALTH

> **" Your medicine is in you and you do not observe it.
> Your illness is from you and you do not recognise it. "**
> Hazrat Ali

Shiatsu can reduce stress and help people feel more relaxed, thereby generally improving their health and quality of life. However giving Shiatsu to someone who still continues with a lifestyle that weakens or damages health is like trying to fill a bucket with a hole in it.

Self responsibility

It is vital for people to learn to help themselves to recognise and accept individual responsibility for their health. We are living in conditions of increasing stress and pollution and the strain of this tells on our well-being. In seeking to counter these conditions we need to examine and understand ourselves and our needs, how we function and our situation in life. Ultimately it is each person's assumption of self responsibility for their healing and growth processes that is important for creating and maintaining health.

The three areas of life that *all* of us can take more responsibility for are diet, exercise and the use of our thoughts and feelings. When people begin to make beneficial changes in any or all of these areas while at the same time receiving regular Shiatsu they start to make great progress towards inner harmony and wholeness.

If you give Shiatsu it is essential that you maintain your own health condition and keep it strong and balanced.

It is useful for you to be able to advise and encourage whoever you give Shiatsu to of the ways by which they can maintain and improve their health.

The influence of diet

A person's diet and way of eating is highly individual, and eating patterns are intrinsically bound up with childhood development and conditioning. They can be remarkably hard to change. The choice of food and the way a person eats both affects and reflects Ki balance and channel functioning in the body.

Food is our basic building block and the quality, type and amount that we eat to a large extent eventually determines our health. 'You are what you eat' is commonly expressed, but even more fundamental is how our bodies digest and use the food. This is directly affected by our moods, emotions and thoughts with the digestive system being especially vulnerable to negative mental attitudes, fear and stress. Tension can often cause good food to be poorly assimilated and make elimination faulty. It can create toxicity in the system. Conversely inadequate and poor quality food can be transformed by the positive functioning of our minds and to some extent be made to satisfy our nutritional need.

Most people are aware of the need to eat in moderation and avoid junk food. However nutrition is a complex area and it can become confusing with many different and sometimes contradictory approaches.

A comprehensive study and common sense are needed to gain clarity and understanding for yourself.

Exercise for health

We thrive on movement. Without it our joints stiffen, muscles weaken, circulation slows, the elimination of waste becomes sluggish, we tend to get fat and age faster.

There are many types of exercise and many reasons for doing them. The Western attitude to exercise tends to be competitive and forceful – we push ourselves into pain, for example, as in aerobics and bodybuilding. The Eastern approach is softer and emphasises stretching and flexibility, as in yoga.

When you exercise for health the aim is to balance mind and body and to promote the ability to relax deeply. What is happening internally whilst doing the exercise is more important than the perfection of form.

How to exercise

Develop an exercise programme to suit yourself and strengthen your weaknesses. Over the weeks suppleness will slowly grow and health and wellbeing improve, as well as the ability to be able to relax more easily in daily life.

The complementary aspect of movement is relaxation. Take a few minutes to centre yourself before beginning to exercise and always relax deeply for at least 5 minutes afterwards by lying flat on your back. In this way you will gain the full benefits of exercising.

Things to remember

- **Exercise regularly.** Only in this way will you see results.

- **Work slowly** and don't force it. Only move and stretch according to your ability.

- **Be centered** and move from your hara (see page 28).

- **Remember to breathe!** – often we unconsciously hold our breath in a stretch.

- **Relax into the stretch.** Suppleness is not achieved through force but by relaxation.

- **Stretch on the outbreath.** Your body can more easily let go.

- **Keep inner attention.** Don't let your mind wander. Concentrate on your physical movements.

- **Use your thoughts** and visualise yourself moving with ease and flexibility. Ask your body to cooperate.

- **Be observant** of your own tensions and body imbalances. Become aware of the feeling of letting go and deeply relaxing.

Channel exercises

The aim of these exercises is to loosen the body and stretch and stimulate the channels. Be aware of any movement of Ki as you exercise. This can be felt physically as sensations such as tingling and heat and will often feel like a release which eases tightness and pain. For full effect do the exercises in the sequence shown, as this follows the natural order of Ki flow in the channels according to the understanding of Oriental medicine.

Repeat all the movements 2 or 3 times.

1 For directing vessels and governing vessels

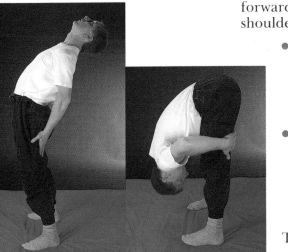

Stand with your feet slightly apart.

- Visualise and move your hara forward as you lean your shoulders back.

  - Place your palms on the back of your thighs for support and let your head tilt back. Don't over-extend.

  - Hold the position. Breathe keeping your hips relaxed and knees soft and feel the stretch along the front of your body.

Then bend forward:

- Imagine your hara sinking back towards your spine.

- Let your head hang down and hold the back of your thighs.

- Breathe and relax into the stretch, feeling it down the length of your back.

Hold and then straighten and relax.

2 For lung and large intestine channels

Stand with your feet a good shoulder width apart.

- Straighten your arms behind your back and interlock your thumbs with your palms facing backwards.

- Spread your fingers to point in opposite directions. Stretch your thumbs and bend forward with straight legs as you exhale.

- Keep your elbows straight and stretch your arms over your head.

- Breathe in the position and hold for as long as is comfortable.

- Feel the stretch especially on the inbreath.

Straighten and relax.

- Then step forward onto one foot keeping the toes of your back foot on the ground for support.

- Inhale as you do this and extend your arms upwards and outwards, opening your hands and stretching your fingers. Look upwards.

- Hold the stretch while holding your breath.

- Step back, relaxing your arms.

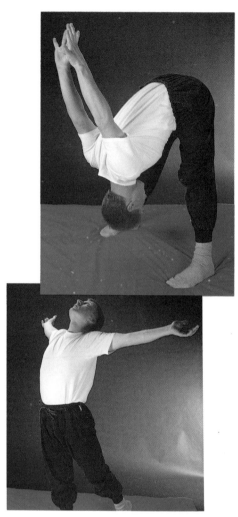

Repeat the sequence with your other foot.

3 Stomach and spleen channels

Kneel and sit back between your heels keeping your toes together.

- Slowly lean back onto your elbows and let your knees part slightly.

If this is enough stretch, hold in this position and breathe.

- For a greater stretch carefully lean right back and rest your shoulders and back on the floor.

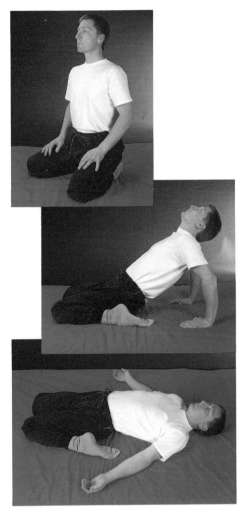

hands. Do this stretch once.

WARNING: Avoid this if you have a bad back.

4 Heart and small intestine channels

- Sit on the floor with your knees bent and the soles of your feet together.

- Hold around your toes, with your feet as close in to you as possible.

- Exhale and bend forward to bring your head towards your toes. Let your elbows move out to the side. (Eventually your knees and elbows will touch the floor, don't worry if they don't yet reach!)

- Hold your maximum stretch with minimum effort and breathe.

Slowly sit up.

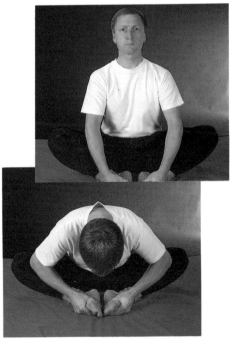

- If this feels comfortable stretch your arms over your head.

- Interlace your fingers with palms facing your head.

- Turn your palms upwards to further increase the stretch. To begin with your knees may lift off the ground and spread. As you gain flexibility begin to keep them together. Remain in the stretch for as long as it is comfortable and breathe.

Slowly come up by supporting yourself with your elbows and

5 Kidney and bladder channels

Sit on the floor with straight legs, heels touching and toes falling out.

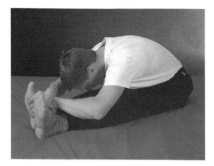

- Fold forward, stretching over your thighs without bending your knees.

- Face your palms forwards and hold the instep of both feet, thumbs pointing towards your heels.

- Bend your head towards your knees. Keep your elbows soft and shoulders relaxed.

- Hold and feel any tightness down the back of your body. On each outbreath relax and sink into the stretch.

Slowly sit up and relax.

6 Heart protector and triple heater channels

Sit on a small cushion in lotus, half lotus or crossed legged position. Make sure you are comfortable.

- Cross your arms and place your hands on opposite knees.

- Exhale as you bend forward. Pull yourself down, let your back bend and head drop.

- Hold the stretch, relax your effort and breathe.

Slowly sit up.

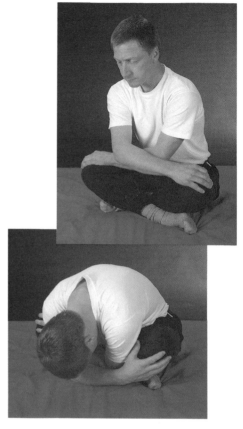

7 Liver and gall bladder channels

Sit on the floor with both legs straight and spread wide.

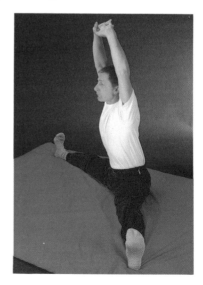

- Keep the back of your knees on the ground and stretch your arms up over your head, clasp your hands and turn your palms upwards. Straighten your elbows.

- Exhale and bend over to one side, taking your hands towards your foot. Keep facing forward and stretch the side of your body.

- Hold the stretch as you breathe and relax into it.

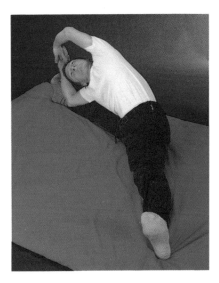

Repeat on the other side.
Slowly straighten and relax.

The effect of thought and emotions

We are not yet fully aware of the tremendous power we are all able to wield through our minds. The degree to which our thoughts and emotions affect the functioning of every cell in our body is hardly realised by most people. Not only do they influence our bodies physically towards health or sickness, but they attract conditions and situations in life, both good and bad. In other words, our thoughts are creative.

To appreciate this fully is the beginning of accepting responsibility for yourself, how you are and what happens to you.

The events of life begin to condition us from the moment of birth and even in the womb. In time this conditioning dulls our awareness and allows us to function in an increasingly mechanical way. The difficulty is that it is hard for us to see this, as we let our own thought patterns and emotional attitudes habitually repeat themselves at an unconscious level. These often tend to be negative, affecting us accordingly, and in our ignorance we blame others and outside things for the resulting adverse situations.

Positive thought is often talked about and even when we sincerely practise this our lives and health may still remain problematic because we fail to take account of our hidden negative ways.

It is essential for each of us to awaken to this whole *unconscious* world of activity that relentlessly continues unnoticed inside us. Awareness brings choice and when we clearly see the way in which our mental activity directly affects our lives we may be in a position to choose life enhancing behaviour instead of destructive patterns.

8

SHIATSU THEORY

> **❝** *Existence is beyond the power of words to define.* **❞**
> Lau Tzu

Shiatsu is based on the concepts and theories of acupuncture and Oriental medicine, which originated in China over 4000 years ago. All natural phenomena are understood to be formed from life energy or Ki, which itself is basically divided into two complimentary forces, Yin and Yang. As this primary energy radiates outwards, it is defined by the 'Five Elements': Wood, Fire, Earth, Metal and Water. From this is created the infinite variety and complexity of all physical manifestations and life as we perceive it.

'TAO' SOURCE → KI → YIN → Wood / Fire, YANG → Earth / Metal / Water → ALL ASPECTS OF LIFE

The holistic concept of Oriental medicine

Central to the understanding of Oriental medicine is the 'holistic' concept of 'oneness'. All of life is seen as sharing the same elements and to be functioning under the same natural laws. Whether it is the life of the Universe or the life of an individual the importance of all things is equally acknowledged as being indispensable to the functioning of the whole.

This means that during illness the complete person should be treated. One part cannot be singled out for attention without regard for its relationship to and the effect it has on all things. The Oriental doctor is concerned with the totality of an individual's physiology and psychology.

He observes all the characteristics and symptoms of a person and from this the form of the treatment emerges. The disease is not even labelled as a specific entity because all illness is seen as coming from the same source – an imbalance of life energy or Ki throughout the body. Consequently conditions of ill health are described by their quality and character, using terms such as Damp, Dry, Heat, Cold, ascending, descending, Full, Empty and so on.

Preventative care is of prime concern and seems to be the highest form of medicine. Traditionally in China doctors were paid to keep all people well and they did this through skillful diagnosis of an individual based on detailed observation. At the first indications of poor health, they would suggest the necessary alterations in lifestyle and diet to help restore Ki balance. When a person was ill, the doctor was seen to have failed and was not paid.

Ki

The Japanese word for vital energy or life force is Ki and it is this energy that constitutes, maintains and activates all things in the Universe.

Ki can take many forms and it is adaptable to different situations, being at the basis of all functions. It exists in various degrees of condensation: in its extreme forms it creates either dense physical matter or disperses, giving rise to gases and the non-physical aspects of life.

Yin and Yang

The 'Great Ultimate', the 'Tao', is the Law of the Universe and the source of all things, according to Oriental understanding. From the Tao springs existence, which is composed in turn of two opposite but complementary parts of the whole known as Yin and Yang.

These two forces define direction of energy and qualities of activity rather than being material or physical phenomena. The interplay between Yin and Yang is the constant source of all change in the Universe. This give and take relationship is the activity of life itself, forming the neverending process of expansion (Yang) and contraction (Yin) and the continuing cycles of growth and decay, life and death.

The Yin and Yang relationship

1 Yin and Yang are relative conditions, not absolutes

One thing will be Yin relative to something but Yang in relation to something else.

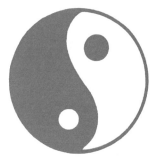

2 One cannot exist without the other

These seemingly opposite forces are complimentary and depend on each other for their existence. Night cannot exist without day and, in the same way, Yin only occurs in relation to Yang.

3 Yin and Yang balance each other

When Yin and Yang fluctuate in more or less their right proportions a state of health is maintained. A relative excess of either creates disharmony.

4 Each can transform into the other

Within each the potential of the other is contained.

Examples of Yin Yang conditions:

YIN	YANG
night	day
moon	sun
dark	light
down	up
contracting	expanding
deep	surface
wet	dry
soft	hard
passive	active
cold	hot
woman	man
negative	positive

Yin, Yang and the body

The functioning of the body pertains to Yin or Yang characteristics, as do all things.

The vital organs and channels are labelled relatively Yin or Yang in quality, and when these function with an overall equal balance between the two forces, health and harmony exist.

This inner balance relates to, and in part is also determined by, a person's relationship to external situations. A balanced life style, in terms of work, diet, exercise, recreation, emotional expression and so on, is needed for well being.

To take an obvious example, too much work (Yang), without sufficient rest (Yin) to balance it, will tire and weaken a person.

The Five Elements

The Five Elements theory, along with Yin and Yang understanding, forms a useful backdrop as to how nature inter-relates with human kind. (Some aspects of Oriental medicine can be better understood with a working knowledge of the Five Elements.) The right interaction of the Five Elements, within the context of free flowing Ki and Yin Yang balance, is seen to bring harmony and order to everything.

Man is an integral part of nature and our internal structure and function mirrors the external order of the Universe. Like the physical world, we wax and wane and follow the yearly seasons and other cycles.

When our lifestyle disregards intrinsic unity and ignores the natural process, inner balance and wellbeing is increasingly lost. The Five Element system is an attempt to classify physical phenomena and give a way in which to understand the Universal processes and laws and how they apply to us.

Five Element division

Five distinct and continuous phases are defined within the perpetually expanding (Yang) and contracting (Yin) activity of Ki.

These divisions are symbolised by the Five Elements of Wood, Fire, Earth, Metal and Water, which relate to the physical composition, cycles and seasons of nature.

These elements need to be understood as *qualities* or processes of nature, rather than as the basic components.

The Five Elements each represent a season in the yearly cycle and have a corresponding type of energy.

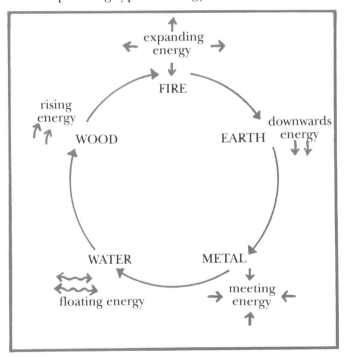

Use of the Five Element theory in diagnosis

Each element is related to different aspects of movement, function, structure, and to the vital organs of the body. They also have an optimum time of functioning (see table on page 120). Any disturbance in any of the Five Elements and their relationship to one another, will affect the physical and psychological balance of a person. This will be observable in subtle ways. For example, in skin colour, sound of voice, emotional tendencies, and so on.

Five element associations

Elements	Wood	Fire	Earth	Metal	Water
Related organ:	Liver/ Gall-bladder	Heart/ Small Intestine	Stomach/ Spleen	Large Intestine/ Lung	Bladder/ Kidney
Colour:	Green	Red	Yellow	White	Blue/black
Sound:	Shouting	Laughing	Singing	Weeping	Groaning
Smell:	Rancid	Scorched	Fragrant	Rotten	Putrid
Taste:	Sour	Bitter	Sweet	Pungent	Salty
Sense Organ:	Eyes	Tongue	Mouth	Nose	Ears
Sense:	Sight	Speech	Taste	Smell	Hearing
System:	Nervous	Circulation	Lymph	Respiration/ Waste	Renal/ Hormone
Tissue:	Sinews/ Tendons	Blood vessels	Muscles/ Flesh	Skin	Bones/ Teeth
Emotion:	Anger	Joy	Pensiveness	Grief	Fear
Climate:	Wind	Heat	Damp	Dry	Cold
Season:	Spring	Summer	Late Summer	Autumn	Winter
Time of Day:	5–10am	10am–3pm	3–7pm	7pm–12mn	12mn–5am

The Five Element cycle

The 'creative' and 'controlling' cycles basically represent the functioning relationships between the vital organs.

The creative cycle

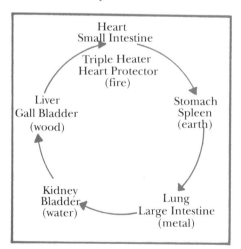

Energy from each organ is passed onto, and 'feeds' the next one, moving in the direction of the arrows.

The controlling cycle

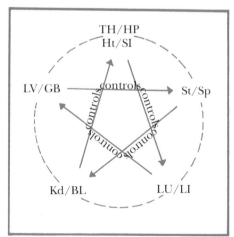

This cycle acts as a balance with each organ being controlled by another.

Five Element theory and Shiatsu

A deep grasp of the Five Element theory and its practical use takes time.

It is something that can be usefully used as you develop your Shiatsu, as a guideline to understanding the relationship between the vital organs and in diagnosing and treating a person.

However, it is not a definitive system and not all conditions will fit neatly into it. There are inconsistencies and, as a model, it is limited when practically applied.

It is best used in a flexible way with other factors also being taken into account.

Channels

Ki flows throughout the body focusing its movement along a network of specific pathways, or channels.

Understanding the channels

Traditionally 14 major channels are emphasised, which govern the functioning of the body and relate to its vital organs, systems and psychology.

Of these, 12 are organ channels named after and relating to specific organs. The two remaining channels, Directing Vessel and Governing Vessel are concerned in a more overall way with Ki balance and regulation in the body.

The channels function individually and they also function as complimentary pairs. This means that the activity in one of the pairs will affect the condition of the other.

The channels also connect to and are influenced by the Five Elements and each of the paired channels manifest the characteristics and attributes of their related element (see table opposite).

The 12 organ channels mirror themselves, each with 2 branches which flow either side of the body. Directing Vessel and Governing Vessel are single and circulate the midline of the body. Channels are not physical structures and they are not visible to the physical eye. However, Ki movement in them can be felt with experience and a developed sensitivity. Changes in the skin's electrical resistance can be measured showing the existence of pathways of energy (channels) with points of accumulation (tsubos). The electric accupuncture machine also works by being sensitive to the measurable changes in the skin's electrical resistance.

Channel diagnosis

In Shiatsu, the vital organs and their function are not viewed only in a physical and anatomical way. They are seen to encompass this and more: the *energy* of the internal organs, flowing in their related channels, are interdependent and operate together (see Five Elements cycle, page 120). They have specific characteristics including emotional and psychological aspects. Consequently, organs have attributes which affect the different systems, functions and structures of the body.

This means that Ki imbalance in one of the channels, felt as stiffness or pain, does not necessarily indicate trouble only in the related organ. Rather, it primarily implies that the organ's energy, its relationship to the whole, is itself out of balance. This can result in a number of different symptoms, as the various related aspects of the body are affected. This of course can also include the organ itself.

Using the channels in a treatment

1 Treat both channels of a pair. They interrelate and affect each other.

2 When working on the limbs, work away from the hara, that is, always towards fingers in the arms and toes in the legs.

3 Press along the length of the channel(s) which pass through a problem area. Ki flow will be stimulated along the channel. This can affect change in areas even when they are not directly touched. This is very useful in treating parts of the body too painful to touch.

4 Working on an area on one side of the body can affect the similar area on the other side. This is true side to side, due to the channels mirroring themselves. There is also a reciprocal relationship in the body, between front and back, top and bottom, and diagonal opposites.

5 There is also a ripple effect in Ki flow and stimulation of one channel will, to an extent, influence Ki balance in the other channels.

Tsubos

Tsubos are points situated along the channels where Ki gathers and is more active and accessible to outside influence. They can be thought of as being like small containers of energy, which, when pressed, open out and release the accumulated Ki, stimulating the flow throughout the body. In Shiatsu and Acupuncture more than 700 tsubos are recognised, although only a fraction of these are commonly used in Shiatsu.

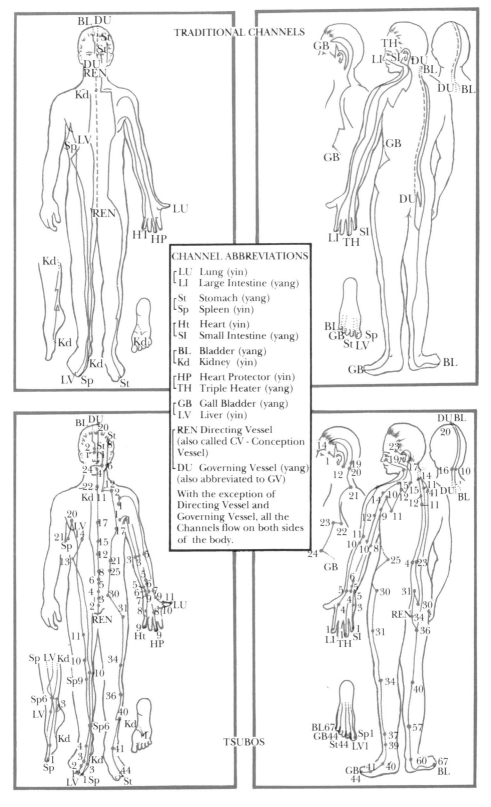

TRADITIONAL CHANNELS

CHANNEL ABBREVIATIONS

LU Lung (yin)
LI Large Intestine (yang)

St Stomach (yang)
Sp Spleen (yin)

Ht Heart (yin)
SI Small Intestine (yang)

BL Bladder (yang)
Kd Kidney (yin)

HP Heart Protector (yin)
TH Triple Heater (yang)

GB Gall Bladder (yang)
LV Liver (yin)

REN Directing Vessel
(also called CV - Conception Vessel)

DU Governing Vessel (yang)
(also abbreviated to GV)

With the exception of Directing Vessel and Governing Vessel, all the Channels flow on both sides of the body.

TSUBOS

Tsubo pressure

Pressure must be given to a tsubo with awareness, beginning gently and only slowly increasing as its resistance gives way and it opens up, allowing a deep penetration. This will activate Ki flow. Pressing too sharply and too quickly will tense and close the tsubo restricting Ki movement.

Using the tsubos

Each tsubo has a specific affect on Ki balance and organ function. In Acupuncture they are exactly located and used in precise combination, depending on the condition being treated. Shiatsu tends to have a broader approach than this and will often emphasise treating the channels by stretching and giving pressure. In this way tsubos are also automatically stimulated. However, some Shiatsu approaches primarily work with tsubos, and use them in an exact way to treat Ki imbalance and sickness.

Finding tsubos

Tsubos are exactly located although there is some individual variation from person to person. They conveniently lie between muscles, bones or in a slight hollow. Acupuncture depends on precise positioning of the needles for effective results. In Shiatsu your overall touch and work on the channels will stimulate the tsubos generally. Specific points can be pressed, but as a beginner do not unduly about their accurate location. You will come to know this in time. As you work, you will very often instinctively press the right spots and the reaction of your partner will also guide you.

Kyo and jitsu

Energy imbalance in the channels is described in terms of it being deficient (kyo) or in excess (jitsu). Kyo and jitsu conditions are relative to each other and depletion of Ki in one area will create an over activity in another. Kyo jitsu interplay within the channels will reflect in the overall impression of **empty** lifelessness (kyo) or tense **fullness** (jitsu) in the body.

Ki imbalance in the channels will manifest itself in different parts of the body, for example, the left side can be kyo relative to a jitsu right side, the lower back can be sunken and kyo compared to a protruding jitsu upper back condition.

The conditions of kyo and jitsu will also be manifest in emotional expression and psychological attitudes and behaviour.

Qualities of kyo

- It contains little or no activity.

- Kyo condition feels hollow and empty of energy, soft to touch and may appear sunken.

- It is a needy, unsatisfied condition which is deepseated and usually hidden.

- Kyo can be thought of a 'low pressure' and it can be the underlying cause of a jitsu condition elsewhere.

- Chronic Kyo condition will change to become brittle and stiff (yet empty).

Qualities of jitsu

- Jitsu can be thought of as the symptoms, the reaction to and compensation for the emptiness of kyo.

- It has a feeling of fullness, being hard and resistant to touch and it can be thought of as 'high pressure'.

- Jitsu is a surface active condition and as such it protrudes and is relatively obvious and visible.

- Jitsu will seek to protect kyo.

Treating kyo and jitsu

The body naturally seeks to balance itself. Ki is in constant flux and movement. At any moment aspects of energy are relatively kyo or jitsu. Problems and sickness only manifest themselves when imbalance becomes fixed and established.

The essential aim of Shiatsu is to assist the body in re-establishing and maintaining its natural state of Ki balance, in other words, health. In giving Shiatsu, discovering kyo and jitsu is fundamental to determining how you treat your partner.

Tonifying kyo

The basic principle is to strengthen or 'tonify' the depleted kyo condition. This is done slowly by holding and giving gradual pressure which penetrates and energises. Wait with patience for Ki to be drawn to fill the kyo emptiness. This cannot be hurried or forced.

Tonifying kyo will affect the whole body.

Dispersing jitsu

On the other hand, a jitsu condition needs to be dispersed. Vigorous techniques such as rubbing, kneading stretching and shaking will help move Ki and reduce congestion.

Dispersing jitsu will affect the local body area.

Finding kyo and jitsu

An easy way to assess a person's general body pattern of kyo and jitsu is to shake a plain sheet and let it naturally fall over them as they lie on the floor. Wait for it to settle. Then notice which areas protrude (jitsu) and which areas are sunken (kyo).

9
A WORD ON DIAGNOSIS

> **&& ** *We must admit that what is closest to us is the very thing that we know least about although it seems to be the thing we know best of all.*
>
> C. G. Jung **&&**

To some extent Shiatsu works anyway, whether you study and learn it in detail or simply give treatments for enjoyment. However if you want your Shiatsu to become increasingly effective and your sensitivity and perception to develop, the understanding and application of diagnosis becomes relevant and necessary.

The possibility of diagnosing a person simply by observing them, listening to them or touching them may seem far fetched.

In fact we quite unconsciously do this in everyday life. Instinctively we 'read' a person to know what they are like. For example, to survive we must know who will hurt us and who we can trust; in choosing a friend or business partner, it is important to assess their quality, reliability, health and so on.

Understanding diagnosis

The intricacies and patterns repeated throughout nature are also mirrored in us. Our bodies are shaped by what is not seen and they reflect and display the whole of our history and condition, physically, emotionally, psychologically and spiritually.

That which takes place internally in us is also revealed on the outside of our bodies. Nobody needs a special talent or to be psychic to be able to attune to this. We only need a little more awareness and practice in reading the signs.

A new approach

Instead of focusing only on a person's problem and what is wrong, diagnosis, or clear observation, can give you the means to see and accept a person as she is. From this point her needs, and the means by which you can nourish and support her, become clear.

In Shiatsu a nurturing quality and attitude is all important. There must be no barriers if real exchange of energy is to take place between two people. When this happens much is revealed and the faculty of intuition is opened.

Fundamentals of diagnosis

Developing perception

Understanding and insight cannot be given to you by someone else. It is only through the practice of observing, touching, asking questions and being open to people and situations that your discernment and intuition will develop. Use every opportunity in daily life to watch people; for instance, how they move, speak, sit, their favourite foods, colours, activities, their expressions and mannerisms.

Keep your mind open. Be nonjudgemental. Let impressions come to you. Don't analyse or look for conclusions. In this way your perception, intuition and understanding of people will develop.

Condition and constitution

There are two principal areas of diagnosis. These are concerned with a person's condition and with their constitution.

The **condition** of a person is directly influenced by, and is a result of, their lifestyle: habits of eating, thinking and activity. The environmental factors, such as pollution, that they are exposed to are also important.

On the other hand **constitutional** tendencies are deep seated and are with everyone from birth.

It is important to gain insight into a person's constitutional disposition as there is always the possibility of preventing undesirable tendencies from becoming symptoms and disease.

Ways of diagnosing

Diagnosis is based on information about a person, which is gathered in different ways:

- **By observation**, noticing such things as skin colour and discolouration, rashes, marks, posture, behaviour.

- **By touching**, which gives you direct information about skin condition, muscle tone, flexibility, areas of pain, lumps and so on. Also you will directly connect with, and feel the quality of, a person's Ki energy.

- **By sensing**, which means using the faculties of hearing, smelling and intuition to gain information, for example from the sound of a person's voice or noticeable breath and body odour.

Diagnostic 'tools'

Specific theories and techniques can also help and guide your diagnosis. The body is full of signs and indications which reflect its history and internal condition of balance.

Many systems of diagnosis have been developed and used successfully over thousands of years.

Hara diagnosis

The different points in the hara will be either relatively empty (kyo) or full (jitsu) of energy (see page 24). Feel for this with your fingertips and without 'trying'; let your whole self be open and sensitive to these differences.

Tuning into the subtle variations of energy in the hara requires patience and practice. You need to be still and centred. Let your hands work together, the resting hand 'listening' as you explore the area with your active hand. Slowly your sensitivity and awareness of the different qualities of Ki will develop. The relatively tight jitsu points are more obvious. Remember that kyo is often concealed and hard to find. Relate what you find to the diagnostic areas of the hara, and also to the channels running through the area. In this way you can achieve a clearer understanding of your partner's condition and treat her accordingly.

You can diagnose the hara both at the beginning of a treatment and at the end to see what changes have taken place.

Hara map

The hara is a person's centre of energy and as such it reflects the condition of the whole body. Like the feet, the hara has areas relating to the organs and systems of the body.

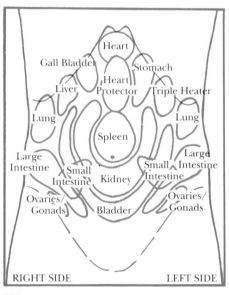

RIGHT SIDE   LEFT SIDE

Ways to diagnose

1 Upper and lower hara

Sit facing your partner and rest the palm of one hand below her navel and the other above and feel for kyo and jitsu. Most commonly you will find the lower part of the hara will be weak and kyo. Tonify the kyo area giving slow and steady penetrating pressure. This will encourage your partner to relax and open and also encourage the jitsu area to soften as Ki is drawn to kyo. In this way the jitsu areas will be able to receive deeper pressure.

2 Compare each side of the hara

Of the two halves on either side of the mid-line of the body, one may be relatively kyo. Tonify this area, using your whole hand to give steady pressure.

You can also use your fingertips to feel the points that correspond to the internal organs mirroring each other either side of the mid-line. Compare how they feel and decide which is the more jitsu. Then tonify the kyo side with steady pressure until you feel the point open and Ki balance between your two hands.

3 Reading the hara map

Sit at hip level close to your partner and face her head, with your hand resting over her navel. Use the first two fingers of your other hand to test hara diagnosis points for their relative kyo (empty) and jitsu (full) condition (see the hara map). Begin with centre top, the heart area, and work down each side under the ribs and then down the centre line to the navel. Change your support hand and use your other hand to test the areas of the lower hara.

Treat the kyo to encourage dispersion of excess Ki in the jitsu points towards these areas.

Test the areas again to see what change has taken place.

Back diagnosis

Back diagnosis will tell you about the chronic weaknesses of a person and what lies behind a problem.

Related areas of the back

The back can be viewed from a broad perspective with areas relating to the vital organs.

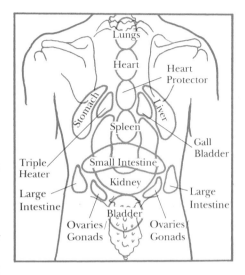

Associated points

Also called Yu points, these are situated along the inner Bladder Channel next to the vertebrae. They relate to and reflect imbalances in the vital organs of the body.

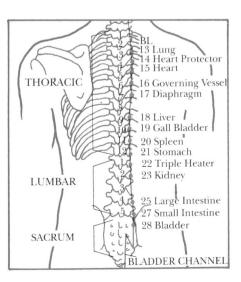

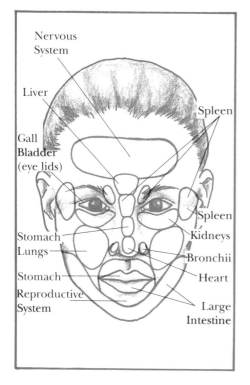

Face diagnosis

The different areas of the face also relate to the organs and systems of the body. Skin colour, tone, texture, the position of marks, spots, wrinkles and the accumulation of fluid all can indicate the condition in the related parts of the body. When these signs are heeded and a person's lifestyle is adjusted to address the tendencies of imbalance, major health problems can be avoided.

Diagnostic areas of the tongue

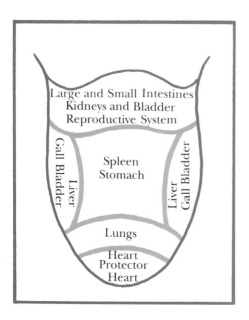

Diagnosis can also be made observing:

- Conditions of channels and tsubos (see pages 121–124).

- Condition of kyo and jitsu in the body (see pages 124–125).

- Yin, Yang and Five Elements classification (see pages 117–121).

- Body posture and movement.

Each of these areas of diagnosis is involved and requires study to master in depth. Knowledge of any will enhance your Shiatsu.

Things to remember

- Observe with an open mind.

- Look for strengths and tendencies.

- Maintain a holistic approach. Strive to see more, not less and the inter-relationship of the whole.

- Continually seek confirmation or contradiction in your assessment. Remain flexible and willing to adjust your opinions as necessary.

- See the overall picture and from this move to noticing detail.

Initially observe with unfocused eyes. See which broad areas jump out and which disappear before looking at specific parts.

- Look for the underlying cause of a situation. That which is obvious may be misleading.

- Notice rashes, discolouration, areas of stiffness and pain in relationship to channels that pass through or near them.

- Observe people in their daily activity when they will be more natural.

10
WIDER ISSUES

The path of self development

Shiatsu can be a catalyst for your own awakening and inner growth. You can change simply by doing it. This may sound strange since, in practising Shiatsu, you focus on the other person and seek to help them rather than yourself. Yet the Shiatsu system of understanding is extensive and, as must now be apparent, in learning about others you are in fact learning about yourself – the very wonderful and specific functioning of your body, mind and spirit and your relationship to other people, society, nature and the universe.

Even more significant is the aspect of 'giving'. Shiatsu is a two-way activity and in giving you also receive, as anyone who practises will tell you. The giving must be done freely as a genuine response and as a deep sharing of yourself, without thought of reward or gain. When this happens, a person's compassion and feeling is opened, and this, along with knowledge and understanding, will eventually begin in them a natural transformation process and the development of their consciousness.

Working on yourself

As you continue to study and practise Shiatsu you may naturally begin to apply its body of knowledge to yourself in a practical way.

Changes can be made in your lifestyle. Your diet may need adjusting, regular exercise taken up and techniques of relaxation and meditation practised. As this happens you will begin to look, feel and be healthier and be in a better position to help others.

Self development exercises

Thinking, reading and gathering information does not develop your consciousness. Knowledge can help awaken you to new possibilities, but it is the actual 'doing' of meditation and exercises that begins an inner transformation. These have to be practised regularly for change to take place.

By experiencing the following exercises for yourself you will be able to recommend them to people who come to you for Shiatsu.

Grounding exercises

1 Hara and feet triangle

time: 10 mins or more

- Stand with your feet shoulder width apart.

- Put your awareness in your hara (3 finger widths down from your navel). Try to get a feeling contact.

- Now imagine a flow of energy down your right leg to the sole of your foot.

- Next, imagine the energy flowing to the sole of your left foot. Take time to feel a contact.

- Then imagine the energy flowing up your left leg back to your hara.

- Continue circulating in this way with your awareness. Form a triangle from your hara→ right foot→ left foot→ hara.

- Move slowly and finish at your hara.

2 Rocking

Place your awareness at your sacrum, weight balanced evenly between both feet.

- Step one foot forward, knees slightly bent.

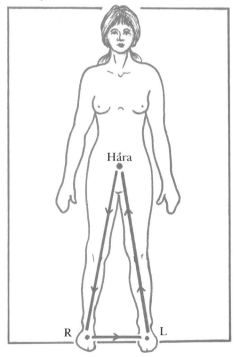

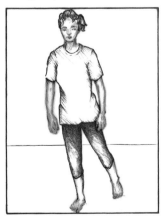

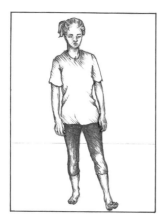

- Bring your weight onto the forward foot. Keep the toes of the back foot on the ground for support.

- Breathe in after you rock forward.

- Then rock your weight onto the back foot keeping the heel of the forward foot on the ground for support.

- Breathe out after you rock back.

- Rock forwards and backwards in this way for 5 minutes, moving slowly.

- Now balance yourself evenly on both feet again.

- Repeat the above procedure with the other foot forward.

- Then balance yourself evenly on both feet and release.

Hara strengthening exercises

1 Stretch pose

time: 1–3 mins

- Lie flat on your back with arms by your side and palms facing down.

- Keep your legs straight, toes pointed, and lift your legs, arms and feet a few inches off the ground.

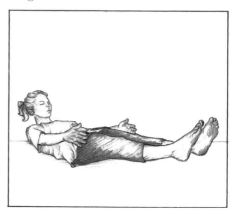

- Look at your toes as you breathe strongly through your nose in short fast breaths.

- Emphasise your out breath as though you are trying to blow a feather from the tip of your nose. Allow the in breath to take care of itself.

- Feel your back pressed into the ground. Try to relax your hara so that it moves with the breath.

- Centre your awareness in your hara as you hold the position.

- Before relaxing hold your last in breath – and hold and hold and hold . . . . . and then let go and totally relax.

2 Qi gong ('Qi' is a Chinese spelling of Ki)
time: 10 mins

- Stand firmly on both feet shoulder width apart.

- Stretch your arms out in front of you with your hands close together as if they were holding a small ball of Ki energy.

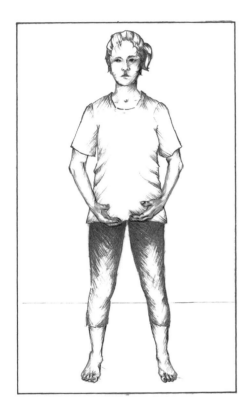

- Breathe in through your nose. Visualise your breath filling your hara.

- As you inhale let your arms widen as though the ball of Ki is expanding between your hands. Open your arms as wide as you comfortably can.

- As you exhale let your arms come together naturally; they should feel as though they 'contain' the small ball of Ki.

- Continue creating a rhythm of breathing and movement and then relax.

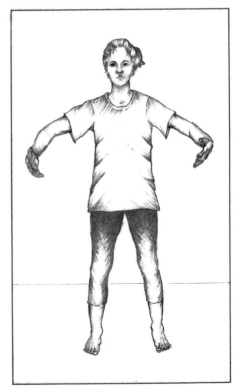

Breathing and relaxing

Use before exercising and when you finish, or at any time.

1 Lie on your back, eyes closed. Centre in your hara and *feel* what it is like to be inside your body.

2 Breathe through your nose (unless it's uncomfortable). Feel the breath come into your body, into your hara and fill you right up to the top of your head and out to your finger tips and toes.

3 Pause for a moment. Then exhale allowing the air gently to go out of your body leaving it soft and empty. On each out breath feel yourself sinking into the ground.

4 Wait, until by reflex action your body breathes in again for itself. In this pause simply 'be' and feel the weight of your body being supported by the ground.

5 Breathe in this way for a while. Then let your breathing take its natural form. Simply lie there and feel yourself in the present.

If you feel discomfort or anxiety during the first part of this exercise, relax and allow your breathing to take any form.

Breathing and relaxation can also be done sitting and even standing. Have your feet shoulder width apart and flat on the floor. Always keep centered and feel your contact with the ground.

Developing your Shiatsu

Shiatsu can be a pleasant pastime or it can be developed to various levels until it becomes a very effective way to prevent sickness and treat ill health. How you use Shiatsu depends upon your individual interest and the amount of effort and time given to its study. If your interest in Shiatsu is for enjoyment, then don't feel intimidated, or obliged to study it further. Giving Shiatsu for fun is a wonderful way to relax with family and friends.

However, what may have started as a casual desire to give massage can, of itself, develop into a more serious interest as the extent of your understanding of Shiatsu and Oriental medicine deepens. At an advanced level the quality of 'being' that you bring to Shiatsu treatments becomes increasingly relevant. The importance of self development is emphasised because your energy affects your partner. In addition to this your own clarity, sensitivity and intuition is needed to guide your perception and insight into her condition. Your treatments are formed from diagnosis and the accuracy of this influences the effectiveness and quality of your Shiatsu. When you work with people in this way, it is essential that you draw from your own experience, and that your advice is appropriate and true. This will only be the case when you are practising what you are talking about.

How to train further

In the West, interest in Shiatsu has exploded over the last few years. In the United Kingdom many very good Shiatsu schools and colleges have been established, offering a high standard of teaching (see page 144 for list and addresses). Visiting Shiatsu experts from all over the world, including Japan, regularly come to the U.K. to teach. Consequently, there is an extensive range and choice of workshops and courses, for beginners, intermediate, advanced students and practitioners.

The formation of the Shiatsu Society (see page 144 for address) in 1981 is largely responsible for the cohesive organisation of Shiatsu interest. It is the non-partisan umbrella organisation for Shiatsu in the UK and the dedication and extensive groundwork of its early members has provided a solid foundation for the development of Shiatsu.

The Shiatsu Society offers a support and information network. It also assesses and guarantees the standard of practice of its members.

For more than just a superficial knowledge of Shiatsu, it is advisable to complete a comprehensive training offered by one of the registered schools. This usually takes place over 3 years and is often divided into 3 stages; beginners, intermediate and advanced. Successful completion of the whole training will give you a diploma which is recognised by the Shiatsu Society. To become a full member of the Shiatsu Society graduates of schools can then meet the Society's assessment panel and be invited onto the Society's register, after demonstrating technical ability, quality of touch and an understanding of the Society's code of ethics.

In America, and other countries of Europe and the world, there is also a fast growing Shiatsu interest and opportunities for training.

And never think that you finish learning Shiatsu. Even as a fully qualified Practitioner, the value of exposing yourself to a variety of teachers and studying different approaches is tremendous. Keep an open, inquisitive and enquiring mind at all times.

APPENDIX I

Chakras and the aura

Ki radiates around each person as an energy field known as the aura. Man is part of the greater Universal energy field, formed of very fine electromagnetic energy which condenses down eventually into the physical forms that we all know well. There is a 2-way movement and Ki energy also emanates out from our bodies, refining its compact physical nature into increasingly subtle vibrations and dimensions.

Energy centres, or chakras, are the link between the physical and the non-physical and act like transformers of Ki. Chakras are situated in the aura and many secondary chakras inter-relate to support 7 major ones. These are located, non physically, along the vertical midline position of the body.

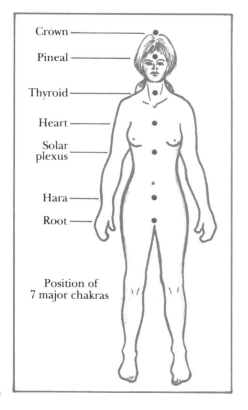

Crown
Pineal
Thyroid
Heart
Solar plexus
Hara
Root

Position of
7 major chakras

Chakras correspond to the glands, organs and characteristics of the body. They also interact and are compatible with channels and the nervous system. Movement of Ki is dependent upon their balanced functioning.

Some people have the ability to see the aura and energy movement. This can be developed through training and can be of value because the aura will indicate the future physical condition of the body, as well as reflecting its present state and past experiences. Science today is beginning to observe the movement of Ki and recognise the importance of our energy fields and their relationship to our existence.

APPENDIX II

Channel extensions

The 14 classical channels of acupuncture traditionally used in Shiatsu only represent part of the network of channels flowing throughout the body.

Shiatsu therapy owes much to the Japanese master, Shizuto Masunaga (1925–81). His system of Shiatsu emphasises the treatment of the whole channel and relates a person's condition primarily to kyo jitsu balance of Ki. Physical manipulation and channel stretches also form an important part of treatment. He also promoted the idea of working along channels from the centre (hara) to the extremities.

In his work he identified extensions of the 12 organ channels. In this diagram the traditional channels are represented by brown lines and the channel extensions by blue lines.

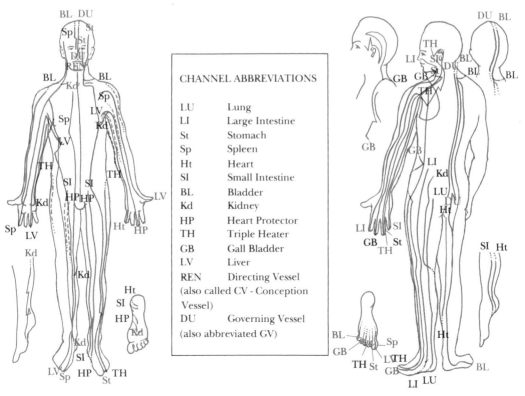

CHANNEL ABBREVIATIONS

LU	Lung
LI	Large Intestine
St	Stomach
Sp	Spleen
Ht	Heart
SI	Small Intestine
BL	Bladder
Kd	Kidney
HP	Heart Protector
TH	Triple Heater
GB	Gall Bladder
LV	Liver
REN	Directing Vessel (also called CV - Conception Vessel)
DU	Governing Vessel (also abbreviated GV)

APPENDIX III

Structures of the body

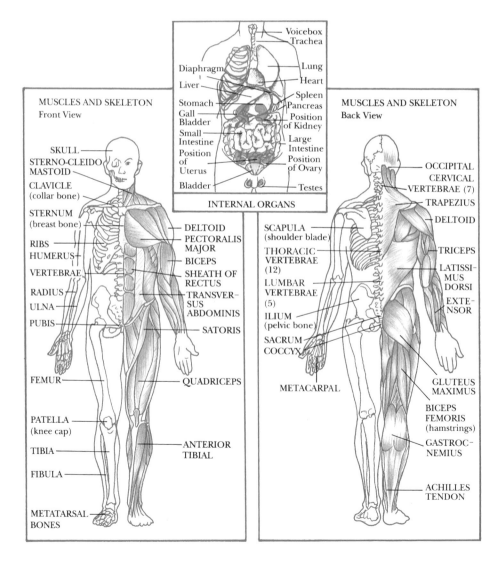

MUSCLES AND SKELETON
Front View

SKULL
STERNO-CLEIDO
MASTOID
CLAVICLE
(collar bone)
STERNUM
(breast bone)
RIBS
HUMERUS
VERTEBRAE
RADIUS
ULNA
PUBIS

FEMUR

PATELLA
(knee cap)
TIBIA
FIBULA

METATARSAL
BONES

DELTOID
PECTORALIS
MAJOR
BICEPS
SHEATH OF
RECTUS
TRANSVER-
SUS
ABDOMINIS
SATORIS

QUADRICEPS

ANTERIOR
TIBIAL

INTERNAL ORGANS

Voicebox
Trachea
Diaphragm
Lung
Liver
Heart
Spleen
Stomach
Pancreas
Gall
Bladder
Position
of Kidney
Small
Intestine
Large
Intestine
Position
of
Uterus
Position
of Ovary
Bladder
Testes

MUSCLES AND SKELETON
Back View

OCCIPITAL
CERVICAL
VERTEBRAE (7)
TRAPEZIUS
DELTOID

SCAPULA
(shoulder blade)
THORACIC
VERTEBRAE
(12)
LUMBAR
VERTEBRAE
(5)
ILIUM
(pelvic bone)
SACRUM
COCCYX

METACARPAL

TRICEPS
LATISSI-
MUS
DORSI
EXTE-
NSOR

GLUTEUS
MAXIMUS
BICEPS
FEMORIS
(hamstrings)
GASTROC-
NEMIUS

ACHILLES
TENDON

APPENDIX IV

Understanding the body

The body is a complex multifaceted organism. Its physical functioning is well documented. Less commonly understood is its psychological significance.

The various parts of the body have emotional characteristics and are susceptible to stress and tension in different ways.

The back

The spine is the supporting element of the body. It relates to uprightness and righteousness of action, mind and spirit. To be said to have 'backbone' denotes a certain character of honour, trustworthiness, courage and sincerity in a person.

The back is the strength area of a person and in danger it is instinctively presented as a shield.

The hips

The hips relate to determination and will. As the shoulders support the head in the upper body, in a corresponding way the hips support the abdomen which connects with self preservation and the natural life of man and woman.

The abdomen

In 4-legged animals the abdomen and hara are protected and covered by the spine and the powerful muscles of the back. But in man, being upright, they are open and exposed. This vulnerability allows for a greater sensitivity and gives us the capacity to feel and relate more intimately with each other.

The belly of a person, the hara, is the primordial source of power and wisdom; gut feelings and the basic drives of sexuality and survival come from here.

Legs and feet

The legs and feet relate to the will to do and act.

The knees are the most prominent joint. They allow a certain grace of movement to the legs and are associated with humility and devotion to a higher aspect. The act of kneeling allows the ego to soften, humble and be receptive to that which is greater, as in prayer.

The feet provide the vital link for the body with the ground and indicate a person's security and confidence of being. They also symbolise direction and a freedom of movement and will.

Arms and hands

The arms and hands act as an extension of the heart. It is through them that love and care can be expressed and the principles of giving and receiving demonstrated. We are able to give out to the world and draw back to ourselves. They are important tools of expression, giving form to our whole range of emotions. With them we are able to grasp opportunities or protect ourselves and keep people at a distance. Feelings of indecision, of being out of control, of being dominated by people or events and unable to take things 'in hand' easily contract the muscles of the arms and hands and inhibit relaxed and easy movement.

Chest

The sturdy protection and support of the ribs is essential, not only physically, but also psychologically and spiritually, as the heart chakra (see page 138) is situated in the chest area. This relates to our emotions and feelings of love and compassion and inspiration. Its very soft nature is easily hurt when our feelings are trampled on and squashed. As a consequence we may try to protect ourselves by hiding our vulnerability and suppressing our true feelings. In doing this, we create deep tensions by cutting off from the true reality of ourselves and feelings such as inferiority, introversion, mistrust and self doubt are created.

The shoulders

The shoulders support, uphold and uplift. It is a willing 'shouldering' of responsibilities, which allows you to give of your services as well as receive from others, that the development of your consciousness can take place.

The neck

The throat chakra (see page 138) relates to expression, and is centered in the neck near the thyroid gland and the voice box. Speech has the potential for tremendous power when it is used freely and in truth. It provides a means to clarify thought and feelings and to develop intelligence and relationships with others. It acts as a bridge between the physical and the spiritual. The neck connects and unites knowledge (the head) with feeling (the heart). In this capacity it will also manifest conflict between the ideas of the mind and the needs of the body.

Head and face

The head is the centre of control and knowledge in a person. It contains 2 major chakras. One is the pineal, which is located in the centre of the forehead and relates to clearseeing, perceiving, intuition and intellect. The other, the crown, is at the centre top of the head. It relates to spirituality and the individual essence of a person. The face relates to beauty and the unfolding of intelligence and feeling. The beauty of the soul can be seen in the eyes and it radiates from the skin. This inner beauty cannot be bought: the way in which we live, think and feel shows on our faces. The eyes reveal the physical, emotional, mental and spiritual condition of a person.

SUGGESTED READING

Zen Shiatsu, Shizuto Masunaga; Japan Publications
Do it Yourself Shiatsu, Wataru Ohashi; Unwin Paperbacks
Shiatsu, the Complete Guide, Chris Jarmey and Gabriel Mojay; Thorsons Publication.
An Introductory Guide to Shiatsu and Oriental Medicine, Chris Jarmey; Thorsons Publication.
Shiatsu, Ray Ridolfi; Optima Books
Shiatsu for Two, Hajo Hadeler; Harbour Publishing Co.
The Book of Massage, Lucy Liddell; Gaia Books
Massage for Common Ailments, Sara Thomas; Gaia Books
Acupressure for Common Ailments, Chris Jarmey and John Tindall; Gaia Books
Zen Imagery Exercises, Shizuto Masunaga; Japan Publications
Chinese Medicine, The Web that has no Weaver, Ted J. Kaptchuk; Rider
Do In, Jean Rofidal; Thornsons
Hara, the Vital Centre of Man, Karl Graf Von Dürckheim; George Allen & Unwin

USEFUL ADDRESSES

The Shiatsu Society
The Administrator
14 Oakdene Road
Redhill
Surrey RH1 6BT
Tel: 0737 767896

There are many registered Shiatsu Schools,
some of which are listed here:

European Shiatsu School
Central Administration
Highbanks
Lockeridge
Wiltshire SN8 4EQ
Tel: 0672 86 362
(classes in London and branches throughout
Britain and Europe)

British School of Shiatsu-Do
188 Old Street
London EC1N 9BP
Tel: 071 251 0831

East Anglian School of Shiatsu
2 Capondale Cottages
New Lane
Holbrook
Ipswich IP9 2RB
Tel: 0473 328061

British School of Oriental Movement
46 Whitton Road
Twickenham TW1 1BS
Tel: 081 744 1974

Bristol School of Shiatsu and Oriental Medicine
81 Cornwall Road
Bishopston
Bristol BS7 8LJ
Tel: 0272 425680/772809

The Shiatsu College
204 Lower Great Lane
Norwich NR2 1EL
Tel: 0603 632555
(classes in London)

Community Health Foundation/Kushi Institute
188 Old Street
London EC1V 9BP
Tel: 071 251 4076

Healing – Shiatsu Education Centre
'The Orchard'
Lower Maescoed
Herefordshire HR2 0HP
Tel: 087387 207

London College of Shiatsu
1 Central Park Lodge
54–58 Bolsover Street
London W1P 7HL
Tel: 071 383 2619

Ki Kai Shiatsu Centre
8 Willow Road
London NW3
Tel: 081 368 9050

The London College of Shiatsu
1 Central Park Lodge
54–58 Bolsover Street
London W1P 7HL
Tel: 071 383 2619

Devon School of Shiatsu
The Coach House
Buckyette Farm
Littlehampton
Totnes
Devon TQ9 6ND
Tel: 080426 593

Hallamshire National Health Centre
10 Dover Road
Hunters Bar
Sheffield S11 8RH
Tel: 0742 662321/346472

Glasgow School of Shiatsu
19 Langside Park
Kilbarchan
Renfrewshire PA10 2EP
Scotland
Tel: 05057 4657

The National Living & Healing Centre
Holistic Centre
Lios Dana
Inch
Annascaul
Co. Kerry
Southern Ireland
Tel: 010 353 6658189

Contact the Shiatsu Society for the Register of Shiatsu Practitioners and Teachers and for a
comprehensive list of recognised Shiatsu schools, colleges and training programmes.